Debra A. Gervais • Tarun Sabharwal
(Editors)

Michael J. Lee • Anthony F. Watkinson
(Series Editors)

Interventional Radiology Procedures in Biopsy and Drainage

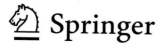

Springer

Editors
Debra A. Gervais
Director of Pediatric Imaging Division
and Associate Director of Abdominal
Imaging and Intervention Division
Massachusetts General Hospital
Boston, MA
USA

Tarun Sabharwal
Consultant Interventional Radiologist
and Honorary Senior Lecturer
Guy's and St. Thomas' Hospital
London
UK

Series Editors
Michael J. Lee
Department of Radiology
Beaumont Hospital
Dublin
Ireland

Anthony F. Watkinson
Nuffield Hospital Exeter
Exeter
UK

ISBN 978-1-84800-898-4   e-ISBN 978-1-84800-899-1
DOI 10.1007/978-1-84800-899-1
Springer London Dordrecht Heidelberg New York

British Library Cataloguing in Publication Data
A catalogue record for this book is available from the British Library

Library of Congress Control Number: 2010937626

Cover design: eStudioCalamar, Figueres/Berlin

Printed on acid-free paper

Springer is part of Springer Science+Business Media (www.springer.com)

Techniques in Interventional Radiology

Other titles in this Series

Handbook of Angioplasty and Stenting Procedures

Transcatheter Embolization and Therapy

Interventional Radiology Techniques in Ablation (forthcoming)

Foreword

It is an honor to write the foreword for this book on biopsy and drainage put together by Drs. Lee and Watkinson. Mike and Tony are well-established experts on intervention and both are renowned for their scientific pursuits and their ability to teach. Their worldwide reputation is acknowledged both in Europe and beyond.

Biopsy and drainage: Perhaps, two of the more underestimated procedures in Interventional Radiology. Why is it that you hear from some interventionalists and even non-interventionalists that, " it is only a biopsy/drainage; no big deal." Actually, both procedures are a "big deal" and should be cultivated and actively pursued by radiologists. Drainage of infected and uninfected fluids may be the best procedure ever invented by radiology. It has stood the test of time, since the first description of the procedure in the mid-1970s. There are two procedures in radiology that can really be called "great." They are arterial embolization and percutaneous abscess drainage. They are great because, when performed correctly, they have an incredibly beneficial effect on a patient's outcome; they have a very high success rate, and there are few contraindications to performing them.

This book also includes discussion on percutaneous biliary drainage, percutaneous nephrostomy, and percutaneous gastrostomy, procedures that are the very core of all interventional radiology. Radiologists should pay careful attention to the chapters on chest drainage and percutaneous gastrostomy and gastro-jejunostomy, as they are both procedures that are underperformed by interventional radiologists. These chapters should help the interventional radiologist become more confident in pursuing these "available" procedures.

The other mainstay of this book is the section on biopsy. Biopsies are the "main stay" of any interventional practice; I believe that all biopsies should be performed by the "interventionalist" in the group, not the radiologist covering ultrasound, CT, or chest for the day. It is only in this manner that the interventional service will grow their biopsy service, and really "push biopsy to the limits" of its capability. More importantly, many newer procedures are a "derivative procedure" of the standard biopsy. Learning basic techniques in ultrasound and CT can only serve the interventional radiologist as he/she learns to perform ablation. Not only do more complicated cases come from the primary physician who refers to you a standard biopsy, but also techniques that one learns in general biopsy can and need to be applied to both simple and difficult ablations. All the biopsy procedures described in this book, will be helpful to the developing and experienced radiologist.

In summary, this book will add to the everyday arsenal of the interventional radiologist. The descriptions, the general writing, and the attention to detail can only serve to enhance your radiology practice.

Peter R. Mueller

Preface from the Series Editors

Interventional radiology treatments now play a major role in many disease processes and continue to mushroom with novel procedures appearing almost, on an yearly basis. Indeed, it is becoming more and more difficult to be an expert in all facets of interventional radiology. The interventional trainee and practising interventional radiologist will have to attend meetings and read extensively to keep up to date. There are many IR textbooks, which are disease specific, but incorporate interventional radiology techniques. These books are important to understand the natural history, epidemiology, pathophysiology, and diagnosis of disease processes. However, a detailed handbook that is technique based is a useful addition to have in the Cath Lab, office, or at home where information can be accessed quickly, before or even during a case. With this in mind we have embarked on a series of books, which will provide technique-specific information on IR procedures. Initially, technique handbooks on angioplasty and stenting, transcatheter embolization, biopsy and drainage, and ablative techniques will comprise the series. In the future, we hope to add books on pediatric and neurointervention.

We have chosen two editors, who are experts in their fields, for each book. One editor is a European and the other is an American so that the knowledge of detailed IR techniques is balanced and representative. We have tried to make the information easy to access using a consistent bullet point format with sections on clinical features, anatomy, tools, patient preparation, technique, aftercare, complications and key points at the end of each chapter.

These technique-specific books will be of benefit to those residents and fellows who are training in interventional radiology and who may be taking subspeciality certificate examinations in interventional radiology. In addition, these books will be of help to most practicing interventional radiologists in academic or private practice. We hope that these books will be left in the interventional lab where they should also be of benefit to ancillary staff, such as radiology technicians, radiographers, or nurses who are specializing in the care of patients referred to interventional radiology.

We hope that you will use these books extensively and that they will be of help during your working IR career.

M.J. Lee
Dublin, Ireland

A.F. Watkinson
Exeter, UK

Preface from the Editors

In preparing *Interventional Radiology Procedures in Biopsy and Drainage* we set out to produce a comprehensive yet concise, portable, and current practical guide to nonvascular interventional radiology procedures suitable for the IR suite. Whether available "on the shelf" in the control room or as a pocket companion, this manual should prove a useful quick reference for physicians in IR training as well as a valuable overview for technologists.

To minimize redundancy, the introductory chapter discusses global issues across the practice of nonvascular IR such as antibiotics and coagulation parameters. While of necessity simplifying these complex topics, which in reality comprise a heterogeneous and variable set of practice patterns across different continents and across different procedures, the chapter provides a general overview and forms a basis for further study. In planning the strategic layout of the manual, we sought international contributions from American, European, and Asian authors to emphasize the universal clinical and technical aspects of nonvascular IR. In keeping with the style of the series, consistent headings across chapters will provide organization for general reading and facilitate rapid fact finding. Each chapter is supported by a short list of up-to-date references that provide a basis for further reading if needed. Selected figures illustrate key concepts.

We thank Professors Lee and Watkinson for their vision and direction in the development of this series. We also appreciate the patience and support of the staff at Springer-Verlag, Melissa Morton, Denise Roland, and Lauren Stoney.

Debra A. Gervais
Boston, MA, USA

Tarun Sabharwal
London, UK

Contents

Contributors

Devrim Akinci MD
Radiology Department,
Hacettepe University School of Medicine,
Ankara, Turkey

Onofrio A. Catalano MD
Abdominal and Interventional Radiology
Department, Massachusetts General
Hospital, Boston, MA, USA

Brian H. Eisner MD
Department of Urology, Massachusetts
General Hospital, Harvard Medical
School, Boston, MA, USA

Nicos I. FotiadisMD, FRCR
Radiology Department, Barts and The
London NHS Trust, London, UK

Afshin Gangi MD, PhD
Radiology/Interventional Radiology
Depatment, University Hospital of
Strasbourg, Strasbourg, France

Debra A. Gervais MD
Pediatric Imaging Division and Abdominal
Imaging and Intervention Division,
Massachusetts General Hospital, Boston,
MA, USA

David J. Grand MD
Department of Diagnostic Imaging,
Warren Alpert School of Medicine, Brown
University and Rhode Island Hospital,
Providence, RI, USA

**Manpreet S Gulati
MBBS, MD, DNB, FRCR**
Department of Radiology,
Queen Elizabeth Hospital & Guy's and St.
Thomas' Hospitals, London, UK

Philip J. Haslam MBBS, MRCP, FRCR
Department of Radiology, Freeman
Hospital, Newcastle-Upon-Tyne, UK

Adam A. Hatzidakis MD
Medical School of Heraklion,
University of Crete, Crete, Greece

Farah Irani MBBS, FRCR
Department of Diagnostic Radiology,
Singapore General Hospital, Singapore

Konstantinos Katsanos MSc, MD
Radiology Department, Patras University
Hospital, School of Medicine,
Patras, Greece

Aoife N. Keeling FFR, RCSI, MRCPI, MSc
Department of Interventional Radiology, Guy's and St. Thomas' NHS Trust, London, UK

William W. Mayo-Smith MD
Department of Diagnostic Imaging, Warren Alpert School of Medicine, Brown University, and Rhode Island Hospital, Providence, RI, USA

Andrew McGrath MB, MRCPI, FFRRCSI
Department of Interventional Radiology, Guy's and St. Thomas' NHS Foundation Trust, London, UK

Melina Pectasides MD
Radiology Department, Massachusetts General Hospital, Boston, MA, USA

Bradley B. Pua MD
Radiology Department, Memorial Sloan-Kettering Cancer Center, New York, NY, USA

Sundeep Punamiya MD, DNB, DMRE
Diagnostic Radiology Department, Tan Tock Seng Hospital, Singapore

Shuvro Roy-Choudhury MBBS, FRCS, FRCR
Radiology Department, Heart of England NHS Foundation Trust, Birmingham, UK

Tarun Sabharwal MBBCh, FRCSI, FRCR
Department of Interventional Radiology, Guy's and St. Thomas' Hospital, London, UK

Anthony E. Samir MD
Abdominal Imaging and Intervention Department, Massachusetts General Hospital, Boston, MA, USA

Ajay K. Singh MD
Department of Radiology, Massachusetts General Hospital, Boston, MA, USA

Stephen B. Solomon MD
Radiology Department, Memorial Sloan-Kettering Cancer Center, New York NY, USA

Alda L. Tam MD, MBA, FRCPC
Section of Interventional Radiology, Division of Diagnostic Imaging, The University of Texas MD Anderson Cancer Center, Houston, TX, USA

Ashraf Thabet MD
Radiology Department, Massachusetts General Hospital, Boston, MA, USA

General Principles of Biopsy and Drainage

Andrew McGrath and Tarun Sabharwal

Modern interventional radiology (IR) techniques and equipment allow image-controlled procedures in most organ systems. The increasing number and complexity of procedures mandates careful patient assessment, close examination of periprocedural factors, and judicious procedure selection to maximize patient benefit and minimize adverse outcomes.

Patient and Procedure Selection

- Decide upon the clinical problem(s) to be addressed by IR
- Diagnostic, therapeutic, or both.

Diagnostic

- Biopsy, aspirate, and diagnostic studies to determine pathologic anatomy/physiology.
- Has the information already been obtained by another method? (e.g., consult all prior imaging studies for evidence of temporal stability of a lesion that might obviate biopsy; results of biopsies in other institutions are often relevant. This may require pursuit of off-site imaging or laboratory studies).

Therapeutic

- Intended outcomes(s)/endpoint(s) of procedure should be explicit from the outset.
- This should involve discussion with the patient's senior clinician and the patient/next of kin (NOK).
- Patient should have accepted in advance the various consequences of the procedure, e.g., indwelling catheter for drainage or long-term feeding/IV therapy

A. McGrath (✉)
Department of Interventional Radiology, Guy's and St. Thomas' NHS Foundation Trust, London, UK

D.A. Gervais and T. Sabharwal (eds.),
Interventional Radiology Procedures in Biopsy and Drainage,
DOI: 10.1007/978-1-84800-899-1_1, © Springer-Verlag London Limited 2011

Consent

- To be obtained by an operator competent to carry out the procedure.
- Obtained from patient or NOK as appropriate.
- Is patient competent to consent? Follow local protocol if not, e.g., consensus of patient's clinicians while informing NOK.
- Parental consent.
- Discuss intended benefits and anticipated risks/adverse outcomes including failure of procedure and requirement to repeat, e.g., nondiagnostic biopsy
- Alternative courses of care and modes of treatment of complications should also be covered.
- Explain intended anesthesia/analgesia and its likely effects including amnesia.
- Ask patient explicitly to voice any concern or questions and to specify any courses of action to which (s)he objects.
- Many interventionalists meet patients well in advance of the procedure, e.g., in a clinic or on a ward. This allows the consent process to be more controlled and is likely to be more satisfactory for all parties; it does, however, take more time.
- Meeting a patient in advance also allows assessment of patient's fitness for procedure, e.g., ability to breath-hold, lie prone, likely cooperation with postprocedural instructions.

Sedation

Benzodiazepines

- IV midazolam, diazepam
- Start with low doses and titrate
- Care in elderly and patients receiving interacting medication

Anesthetic Input for Conscious Sedation

Input from an anesthetist is invaluable in many circumstances, for example:

- Patients with cardiac or respiratory compromise
- Patients with hepatic or renal impairment
- Patients with issues around airway control
- Prolonged procedures which would require high doses of sedation and analgesia
- Patients with previously documented problems with conscious sedation

Patients should be fasting for 4–6 h prior to procedures needing sedation.

Advance assessment by IR and anesthetics can anticipate these problems. Many interventionalists advocate general anesthetic for longer and more complex procedures.

Analgesia

Local

- Lidocaine solution for injection or in jelly preparation
- Bupivicaine for longer onset and duration
- Topical local anesthetic sprays/creams – often ignored but may be useful for skin analgesia

Systemic

- Opioids: fentanyl, morphine, pethidine usually IV or IM
- Paracetamol: IV, PO, or PR
- NSAIDs, e.g., rectal diclofenac

Antibiotics

- Practice varies; IV antibiotic cover is mandatory for any procedure that is intended to or potentially will transgress or instrument a structure that is assumed to be infected, e.g., nephrostomy for pyonephrosis, PTC for biliary sepsis, or abscess drainage. It should be anticipated that these procedures will result in at least a transient bacteraemia.
- Commonly antibiotic therapy will already have been begun by clinicians.
- Some interventionalists use antibiotics routinely for other procedures, e.g., GI intervention, vascular access.
- Follow local guidelines to cover relevant organisms; consult relevant microbiological laboratory reports and local clinical infection services.

Hemostasis

Advance consideration must be given to the likely volume, rate, and duration of bleeding.

Factors Influencing This Include

- Size and number of puncture(s)
- Vascularity of tissue transgressed
- Amount of manipulation of equipment through access route
- Likely effectiveness of manual compression or positional compression

- Use of embolic material to plug site
- Likely patient compliance with postprocedural advice for hemostasis
- Antiplatelet medication, heparins, warfarin, and thrombolytics
- Liver and renal disease, sepsis, massive hemorrhage, and massive blood transfusion
- Heritable coagulation disorders

Procedures May Be Graded into Low, Moderate and Significant Bleeding Risk

Laboratory Values

- Have full blood counts, clotting profiles obtained for all procedures and consider group and save in the more complex or complicated. Most operators use cut-off values of 1.5 for INR and 50,000 for platelet levels.
- Many bleeding tendencies are not necessarily apparent from routine coagulation tests, e.g., low-molecular-weight heparin (LMWH) effects and platelet dysfunction.
- If in doubt seek advice from hematology/coagulation service.

Medication

- Increasing numbers of patients present to IR on antiplatelets and anticoagulants.
- Ideally all these should be discontinued for procedures where hemostasis is problematic, especially biopsies where manual compression is poorly or not effective, e.g., lung, liver, and kidney.
- Cessation of all medications may be problematic especially in patients with recently placed arterial stents (especially drug eluting coronary stents). Careful consideration of risks and benefits by all the relevant clinicians is required in these circumstances; these patients must also be alerted to potentially increased rates of bleeding. Biopsy of regions where direct manual pressure cannot achieve hemostasis may require stricter guidelines than biopsy of areas where direct pressure can be applied.
- Duration of action must be borne in mind, e.g., 4–6 h for unfractionated heparin, days to weeks for some antiplatelet agents.
- Clopidogrel should be stopped for 5 days for moderate risk and clopidogrel and aspirin should be stopped for 5 days for high risk.
- Low–molecular-weight heparin (LMWH) should be stopped for one dose or 24 h.

Embolization

- Embolization, e.g., of gelatin sponge through coaxial needle systems should be *considered* for any procedure where hemostasis is in doubt.
- Some operators routinely embolize all solid organ biopsy sites, others reserve this for focal biopsies involving more instrumentation.

Complications and Management

Ideally, all potential complications should be anticipated

- To facilitate prompt recognition and management.
- To allow patient consent.
- To plan in advance for management by IR, e.g., thoracostomy tube for lung biopsy pneumothorax.
- To allow advance notice if required to relevant clinical service(s) to assist in management of complication(s).
- Nonradiologic information may be useful, e.g., spirometry prior to lung biopsy to help determine risks of pneumothorax or need for admission after biopsy.
- Reversal agents for sedation and analgesia should be easily available in case of respiratory depression.
- IV prehydration for septic/ill patients should be considered (e.g., in biliary drainages to prevent hepato-renal syndrome).

Bleeding: Management

- Assess clinical severity and likely site.
- Apply manual compression if possible – this is often ignored.
- Consider degree of intervention required to stop hemorrhage.
- Consider embolization procedures in solid organs or bowel, covered stents in vascular system.
- Reverse any anticoagulation if necessary and safe to do so, take advice from hematology regarding the administration of coagulation factors.
- Contact relevant clinician including surgical services if surgical management is considered.
- Decide where patient should go – intensive care, ward, or home depending upon severity.

Infection: Management

- Assess clinical severity and likely site – local infection versus systemic sepsis
- Take relevant samples for culture
- Give appropriate antibiotics
- Resuscitate with fluid, oxygen, etc. for acutely ill patient
- Consider IR intervention, e.g., drainage of collection or obstructed system

Unintended Transgression of Organ: Management

- Many organs tolerate puncture surprisingly well.
- Bowel transgression requires close monitoring of abdomen for peritonitis and may require antibiotic administration if a catheter has traversed bowel.

- Injury to pleural space/thorax should be assessed clinically for pneumothorax or intra thoracic hemorrhage, CXR at least is appropriate.
- Injuries likely to bleed, e.g., liver, spleen, kidney, vasculature should be assessed for hemodynamic status and stability.
- For all injuries, full clinical assessment and radiological assessment should be employed as necessary; contrast-enhanced CT is often extremely useful.

Imaging Guidance, Access and Planning

Use most appropriate modality or modalities

- To visualize relevant normal and pathological anatomy and all equipments
- To manage complications
- To which there is access for required time
- Which has relevant staffing for required time
- Which can accommodate required patient monitoring
- To minimize ionizing radiation especially in children and pregnant patients

Many drainages or biopsies of large and superficial lesions can be carried out under ultrasound alone. Use of wires (beyond a single guide wire that can be seen on ultrasound) will often need fluoroscopy and ultrasound (US). Deep lesions and lung and bone lesions usually require CT. Access to a lesion can be obtained under CT and the patient transferred to a fluoroscopy suite with an initial needle or wire in place. US has the advantage over CT of real-time visualization and it does not use ionizing radiation.

Determination of the position of introduced devices in the patient's anatomy is of vital importance. As many methods as necessary should be used to be confident of equipment position including direct visualization on cross-sectional images, conformation of wires and catheters to expected anatomic or pathologic shapes/routes, image guided injection of contrast material, and aspiration of expected material.

Route of access should transgress as few structures as possible. Indwelling hardware must be considered and usually avoided. Likelihood of complication from traversal of various structures is important to consider.

Potential complications of specific routes must be considered:

- Pneumo/hemothorax when traversing pleura, intercostal space, lung
- Hemoperitoneum, retroperitoneal hematoma, subcapsular hematoma: liver, spleen, and kidney
- Pneumoperitoneum, peritonitis traversing bowel/biliary tree
- Hemorrhage traversing vascular structures
- Pancreatitis

Planning with surgical colleagues is appropriate in preoperative biopsies, particularly in the limbs to avoid contamination of specific compartment with malignant cells.

Future use of the access point should be considered, e.g., attitude of gastrostomy puncture for future conversion to trans-gastric jejunostomy, higher calyx puncture if antegrade ureteric stent considered after nephrostomy.

Consider contrast materials to assist access; barium given 24 h prior can show colonic position, excreted iodinated contrast can facilitate puncture of a nondilated renal collecting system under fluoroscopy, the stomach is inflated to puncture for gastrostomy.

Anatomy can be altered to allow easier imaging or safer equipment route. Injection of saline can separate adjacent organs temporarily or alter skin contour to allow more convenient US probe positioning. Iatrogenic pneumothorax can be produced to avoid transgressing lung in mediastinal biopsy.

Equipment must be available prior to starting procedure; if stocks are not routinely maintained, check before starting. Ideally, at least two of each item should be to hand. All required personnel must be on site before the procedure is started; local facilities must be adequate to deal with complications.

More procedures are being carried out as day cases. Prior to a procedure, an assessment of the patient's likely recovery must be made. Ideally, the interventionalist should see the patient.

Factors to consider include:

- Patient's ability to follow postprocedural advice.
- For day procedures patient should ideally be accompanied home and live relatively close to the hospital.
- Likelihood of complications.
- Patient's likely physiologic reserve to tolerate complications or expected outcomes, e.g., postprocedural pain.

Full consideration of these factors can avoid emergency admission after a day case procedure or emergency transfer from ward care to an intensive care setting.

Abscess/Cavity Drainage Tools and Techniques

Direct trocar puncture can be used in large superficial lesions. The trocar may advance farther than intended as the catheter passes through the superficial tissue and, unless the deep surface of the lesion is easily seen in real time, use of a guide wire is probably safer.

21G needles with a 0.018-in. wire can be used when a very narrow access route is available or if avoidance of puncture of surrounding structures is of extreme importance; it is useful also when multiple punctures might have to be carried out before access is gained. The 0.018 in guide wire is not always robust enough to allow the associated 4 Fr dilator to track through tough or fibrotic tissue, e.g., transplant nephrostomy access.

18G needle puncture will accept a 0.035-in. wire. For dilating tracks a stiff wire is useful. Many interventionalists dilate to 1 Fr size larger than the intended drain.

The integrity of the cavity wall should be considered. Despite floppy or curved tips, a friable wall can be transgressed with a wire. It may be useful to form a tighter curve in the stiff part of the wire to help it conform to a small cavity.

Point of access for abscess drainage should allow sideholes to rest in the most dependent part; extra sideholes can be added for long lesions.

The minimum catheter size necessary to allow cavity contents to drain is required. Simple fluid collections may require only 6 or 8 Fr catheters. Smaller catheters are, however, more likely to kink between the skin and the cavity. Complex lesions including pancreatic collections may require up to 20–30 Fr catheters. Multilobed collections may require several catheters simultaneously.

Most smaller bore drains have a pigtail or less often a "mushroom"; larger ones are more often straight. Formation of the pigtail implies that the catheter is free in a fluid space and not misplaced in an adjacent solid structure; it also serves to anchor the drain in place but all drains should be secured to the patient with sutures and/or adhesive dressing.

Unless fluid drains very quickly, most drains should be flushed at least every 24 h with saline to maintain patency; for abscesses this may also help to wash out the lesion. Gravity drainage is most common; suction drainage may be useful, e.g., in cavity sclerosant therapy.

Aspiration to dryness is appropriate for small volumes or those too small to accept a catheter. Aspiration for diagnosis is indicated in collections of uncertain etiology especially if a hematoma is suspected. Leaving a drain in a sterile hematoma may convert it to an abscess and complete drainage is slow and difficult. Many drainage procedures are probably best considered as two part procedures with decision to place a catheter made on the basis of the aspirate. Gross inspection of the aspirate is used; some operators employ microscopy.

Laboratory samples should always be sent; for microbiology and if indicated for cytology. If aspirate yields little material and malignancy is a possibility, a tissue biopsy can be carried out in the same procedure.

Immediately after placing a drain in an abscess, the lesion should be aspirated to dryness as far as possible. Pleural and ascitic drains are allowed to drain freely, or a proportion aspirated immediately.

Before removing a drain, ideally it should be shown that the clinical problem ascribed to the collection has improved or resolved, the rate of drainage of fluid is nil or very small, and that the fluid in the collection has resolved on imaging. Special cases include cholecystostomy tubes, which may be impossible to remove without causing bile peritonitis. Cholecystostomy tubes should be left in situ for 6 weeks to allow a mature track to form before removal.

Biopsy Tools and Techniques

Biopsy samples should be as large as necessary for diagnosis but as small as possible to avoid excess trauma.

Fine needle (22–25G) biopsy is routinely used for thyroid lesions but can be carried out in any lesion. Close cooperation with cytopathology is essential; a cytopathologist on site to determine adequacy of FNA samples is invaluable.

FNA samples are too small to determine subtypes of some lymphomas and surgical excision or large core biopsies are often preferred. Nontargeted liver biopsies require a minimum number of portal triads to be diagnostic. Nontargeted renal biopsies often require a histopathologist on site to determine adequacy of sample.

Core biopsy needles commonly used range from 15 to 20G. Most are partly or fully automated: the inner needle can be advanced manually or automatically and the outer needle is usually automatic. The length of "throw" or how far the needle advances when fired is indicated on the package and should be borne in mind when planning biopsies.

A coring needle can be put through a shorter needle 1–2G sizes larger. This allows multiple samples through one puncture in the organ surface and allows injection of embolic material along the path of the coaxial needle through it as it is withdrawn to plug the puncture site. It can also be exchanged over a wire to allow drain insertion, e.g., into the pleural space.

Samples are sent in formalin or cytological fixing solution. Fresh samples in saline may be required for electron microscopy and other tests. It is vital to consult the relevant laboratory department in advance.

Puncture Site Plugging

For biopsy this requires coaxial access. The biopsies are taken and the outer needle is left in place capped or with the inner needle in place. It must be borne in mind that there is a needle through the capsule of the liver/kidney/spleen and the movement of this with respiration can cause further injury; the coaxial needle should be in place for as short a time as possible. The embolic material should have been prepared before puncture.

The distance between the needle tip and the organ surface and between the needle tip and deeper structures in the organ (vascular lumen, biliary lumen, etc.) is important. Ideally, embolic material will be deposited in the biopsy site and in the parenchyma along the needle path avoiding embolization of material into, e.g., vessels or biliary tree and without depositing any outside the organ.

Collagen plugs are made by rolling cut pieces of the material to produce short cylinders that fit in the outer needle and can be pushed through and out of it with the inner needle or with saline injection. The collagen cylinder size can be checked in the needle bore at the start of the procedure before the puncture is made. Many interventionalists find it easier to control the final position of collagen cylinders than collagen slurry; cylinders may be identified on fluoroscopy by their air contents or if soaked in contrast material. However, they become more difficult to use when wetted.

For biliary procedures a sheath is introduced over the existing wire into the track. Contrast injection allows retraction of the sheath tip until it is no longer in the lumen of any large duct or vessel and sits in liver parenchyma. The wire is removed and collagen cylinders are introduced into the sheath. This can be done by cutting off the hemostatic valve or by loading them into a smaller sheath and introducing this into the larger sheath. The collagen units are then deposited along the track under fluoroscopic guidance, stopping as the sheath tip reaches the capsule.

Conclusion

Key Questions to Address

What is the clinical problem to be addressed?

Is this procedure appropriate to this problem?

Is there a more appropriate alternative course?

For a diagnostic procedure, will its outcome influence patient management?

Have contraindications been considered?

Has all preprocedural imaging and the patient's clinical status been reviewed?

Has an access route been planned?

What is the intended outcome or endpoint of the intervention?

Do all relevant parties (including the patient or next of kin) have an appropriate understanding of the procedure and are relevant clinicians informed and available if necessary?

Have the following been considered in advance: hemostasis, antibiotic therapy, sedation, analgesia, patient preparation, positioning, and anesthesia (including need for admission vs day case), and equipment and staff availability (including access to imaging facility)?

Suggested Reading

1. Patrick CM, Clement JG, Sanjoy K. Consensus guidelines for periprocedural management of coagulation status and hemostasis risk in percutaneous image-guided interventions. *J Vasc Interv Radiol*. 2009;20:S240-S249.
2. Quality Improvement Guidelines for Preventing Wrong Site. Wrong procedure, and wrong person errors: application of the joint commission "universal protocol for preventing wrong site, wrong procedure, wrong person surgery" to the practice of interventional radiology. *J Vasc Interv Radiol*. 2009;20:S256-S262.
3. David K, Iain R. *Interventional Radiology: A Survival Guide*. Philadelphia, PA: Elsevier Churchill Livingstone; 2005. ISBN: 0443100446.
4. Karim V. *Vascular and Interventional Radiology*. Philadelphia, PA: Saunders Elsevier; 2006. ISBN: 0721606210 DDC: 616.1307572 LCC: RD598.5.
5. John AK, Michael JL. *Vascular and Interventional Radiology: The Requisites*. Philadelphia, PA: Mosby; 2004. ISBN: 0815143699 DDC: 617.413059 LCC: RD598.67.

Liver Biopsy

Ashraf Thabet

Clinical Features

- Nonfocal liver biopsy may be required to diagnose or stage diffuse parenchymal disease such as cirrhosis, viral hepatitis, autoimmune hepatitis, primary biliary cirrhosis, primary sclerosing cholangitis, hemachromatosis, and Wilson's disease.
- Focal liver biopsy may be necessary to diagnose or stage primary or secondary hepatic malignancy and to differentiate malignancy from benign hepatic masses such as focal nodular hyperplasia and hepatic adenoma.

Diagnostic Evaluation

Clinical

- Review the patient's history to assess for known diffuse parenchymal liver disease, predisposing factors to or history of malignancy, allergies, medications, patient's ability to cooperate with the procedure, bleeding diathesis, or liver transplantation.
- Review of cardiac and pulmonary history.
- Physical examination:
  — Mental status: Is patient able to give informed consent and follow instructions?
  — Presence of jaundice.
  — Abdominal distention from ascites.

A. Thabet
Radiology Department, Massachusetts General Hospital, Boston, MA, USA

D.A. Gervais and T. Sabharwal (eds.),
Interventional Radiology Procedures in Biopsy and Drainage,
DOI: 10.1007/978-1-84800-899-1_2, © Springer-Verlag London Limited 2011

Laboratory

- Check PT, PTT, INR, and platelet count to assess whether coagulation parameters need correction.
- Elevated alpha-fetal protein may raise the suspicion that a focal lesion represents hepatocellular carcinoma.
- Echinococcal serology if prior imaging is suspicious for hydatid disease; percutaneous aspiration may risk dissemination or anaphylaxis.

Imaging

Use ultrasound or, for focal biopsy, contrast-enhanced CT/MRI to

- Assess need for biopsy: benign masses such as hemangioma may often be diagnosed based on imaging findings alone.
- Exclude biliary dilatation.
- Demonstrate location of the mass and any local and distant spread.
- Plan a safe access route.
- Assess for ascites.

Indications

- Determine nature and extent of diffuse parenchymal disease.
- Differentiate benign from malignant hepatic masses.
- Stage malignancy.
- Obtain material for microbiologic analysis.

Contraindications

- Uncorrectable coagulopathy
- Inability of patient to cooperate
- Lack of safe access to lesion
- Adverse reaction to intravenous contrast if needed
- Hemodynamic or respiratory instability

Alternative Therapies

- Percutaneous biopsy without imaging guidance
- Transjugular liver biopsy

- Open or laparoscopic surgical biopsy
- Endoscopic ultrasound-guided fine-needle aspiration (FNA)

Anatomy

Assess the position of the gallbladder, bowel, pleural space, and dilated bile ducts to avoid inadvertant puncture.

Normal Anatomy

- The right and left lobes of the liver are separated by the middle hepatic vein and gallbladder fossa.
- The pleura extends more inferiorly along the lateral and posterior aspects of the liver.
- The superior epigastric artery courses through the rectus sheath.

Aberrant Anatomy

- The colon may be interposed between the liver and anterior abdominal wall.
- The liver may move cranially as the diaphragm is relaxed when procedural sedation is used.
- The liver may be displaced away from the abdominal wall by ascites.

Equipment

Biopsy Needles

- *Fine needle aspiration (FNA)*: Obtain cells sufficient for cytologic analysis.
  — Any hollow needle (e.g., Chiba, Turner).
  — Typically 20–22G.
- *Core biopsy needle*: Obtain tissue sufficient for histologic analysis.
  — Most commonly used is an automated, spring-activated, side-cutting needle.
  — 18–20G is adequate, although needles as large as 14G may be used, particularly for large hepatic masses or nonfocal biopsy.
  — May be disposable or nondisposable.
- *Coaxial needle*: Typically 11–19G, depending on the size of biopsy needle.

Medication

- *Pain control*: Administer local anesthestic with 1–2% lidocaine.
- *Nausea:* In patients who receive procedural sedation, an antiemetic such as ondansetron may be required.
- *Procedural sedation*: Intraprocedural analgesia and anxiolysis with fentanyl and midazolam is often adequate. Some interventionalists may choose to employ procedural sedation in all biopsy patients or in selected cases where the need for additional anxiety control is anticipated. General anesthesia is rarely required.

Procedure

Ultrasound-Guidance

- Modality of choice for nonfocal liver biopsy (Fig. 1); preferred modality for some focal liver biopsies (Fig. 2).
- Compared to CT, US enables continuous real-time visualization, employs no radiation, is more readily accessible, and has a lower cost. However, intervening bowel and pleural space is difficult to visualize.
- Perform full sonographic examination of the liver, plan access, measure distance, and determine angle of approach.
- Doppler examination can be performed to assess for intervening vessels (e.g., superior epigastric artery, portal vein).
- Biopsy can be performed using free-hand technique with one hand controlling the transducer and one hand manipulating the biopsy needle. Alternatively, a biopsy-needle guide, which attaches to the transducer may be used.

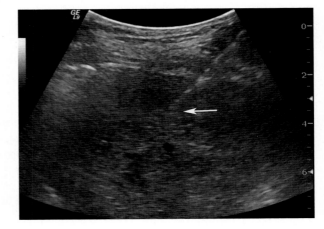

Fig. 1 Ultrasound-guided nonfocal biopsy in a 71-year-old man with hepatitis C and cirrhosis. Coaxial needle (*arrow*) is oriented in a medial to lateral trajectory as it enters the liver

Fig. 2 Ultrasound-guided focal liver biopsy in a 66-year-old woman with hepatitis C and rising serum alpha-fetal protein. (**a**) Preliminary sonogram demonstrates a focal hepatic mass (*arrow*). (**b**) A core biopsy needle (*arrow*) is advanced through the coaxial needle into the hepatic mass. Pathology demonstrated hepatocellular carcinoma

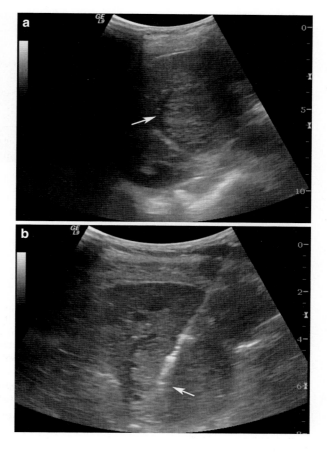

- Needle is best visualized when aligned in the center of the beam along the long axis of the transducer.
- See needle tip as echogenic complex. Visualization of the needle tip is improved when a jiggling "in-and-out" motion of the needle is performed.
- Echogenic needle-tip enhancers are also available but are typically not necessary.

CT Guidance

- Compared to US, CT (Fig. 3) is easier to perform but is associated with longer procedure time, radiation, and higher cost.
- Preferred modality in cases where lesion is not well seen on ultrasound, particularly small, deep lesions. Typically not used for nonfocal liver biopsy.
- A grid is placed on the skin prior to the preliminary CT; position of the grid can be determined based on review of prior imaging.

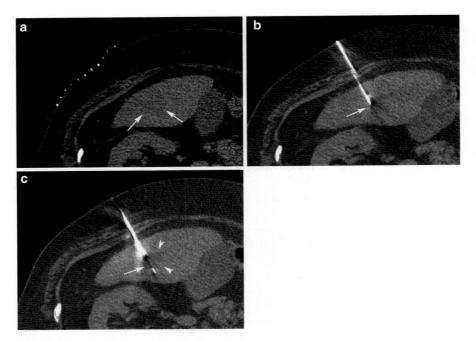

Fig. 3 CT-guided focal liver biopsy in a 73-year-old man who presents with altered mental status, hypercalcemia, and a focal hepatic mass. (**a**) Non-contrast-enhanced CT demonstrates a subtle 5-cm hypodense lesion (*arrows*) in segment 6 of the liver. (**b**) Coaxial needle (*arrow*) is advanced into the periphery of the lesion. (**c**) Inner trochar of the core biopsy needle is advanced into the lesion (*arrowheads*). The specimen chamber (*arrow*) is well seated within the lesion. Pathology revealed metastatic adenocarcinoma of pancreaticobiliary origin

- Obtain preliminary CT of the upper abdomen. Path and distance to lesion can be assessed.
- Obtain CT after each needle adjustment.
- Remove stylet when imaging the coaxial needle to reduce streak artifact that may obscure lesion.
- Real-time visualization of needle placement may be performed with CT fluoroscopy, although this may increase radiation dose.

Planning an Access Route

- A subcostal or subxiphoid approach may reduce risk of pain, pneumothorax, and hemothorax, which some operators believe occur more frequently with an intercostal approach.
- Often, however, an intercostal approach along the mid-axillary line may be required, particularly if procedural sedation is used where the liver may rise cranially.

- If a nonfocal liver biopsy is performed with sonographic guidance, a trajectory pointing away from the gallbladder is preferred to avoid inadvertant injury to the gallbladder.
- For focal liver biopsy, target periphery of lesion to avoid potentially necrotic center that may diminish diagnostic yield.
- *Liver lesions along the diaphragm*:
  — US affords real-time guidance and increased flexibility in needle positioning.
  — If CT is required, a transpleural approach may be necessary. Angling gantry may also be useful.
- *Lesions adjacent to the liver capsule*:
  — Choose an access that provides for intervening normal liver parenchyma between the site of needle entry through liver capsule and lesion.
  — This may reduce the risk of intraperitoneal hemorrhage by providing a tamponading effect.
- *Lesions apparent only on contrast-enhanced CT*:
  — May advance coaxial needle into liver and approximate position of lesion by anatomic landmarks defined on prior imaging.
  — Administer IV contrast and repeat scan; obtain at very least the phase of enhancement when lesion is best seen as indicated on prior examination.
  — Adjust needle position according to lesion location as depicted on contrast-enhanced images.
- *Ascites*:
  — Liver may be displaced away from the abdominal wall, which may make obtaining needle purchase within a lesion challenging. Perform paracentesis, if needed, particularly if moderate or large perihepatic ascites are present.

Technique

- Clean and sterilize skin using standard technique.
- Administer local anesthetic in the subcutaneous tissue.
  — If using ultrasound, apply local anesthetic along the planned biopsy needle path from the skin to the liver capsule using real-time guidance.
- Wait 1 min for anesthetic to take effect.
- Make a 5-mm skin incision using a scalpel blade.
- *Coaxial technique*:
  — Suitable for nonfocal and focal liver biopsy.
  — Minimizes number of passes through liver capsule.
  — Advance coaxial introducer needle into the liver.
  — Through coaxial needle, may obtain fine-needle aspirates and core biopsies.
- *Tandem technique*:
  — Suitable for focal liver biopsy.
  — Place 20–22G needle (e.g., Chiba) into lesion.

— Parallel to this needle, insert second needle (20–22G for FNA or 18–20G for core biopsy) through incision parallel and in tandem to first needle into lesion and obtain specimens.
— 22G needle less suitable for deep lesions as may deflect easily and is more difficult to maneuver while advancing.
- *Fine needle aspiration*:
  — Attach 10-mL syringe to needle.
  — When needle is at periphery of lesion, jiggle needle using a short-stroke "in-and-out" motion while maintaining suction on the syringe of approximately 5 mL.
  — Discontinue suction on syringe before withdrawing needle to prevent aspiration of blood and cells from needle tract.
  — Preserve on glass slides in ethanol or place aspirate directly into methanol-based preservative solution.
- *Core biopsy*:
  — Core biopsy needle systems differ from one manufacturer to another. Familiarize yourself with operation of gun prior to use.
  — Prepare needle by withdrawing inner trochar into outer cannula.
  — Advance needle into lesion.
  — Advance inner trochar into lesion.
  — May reconfirm position of needle tip by US or CT.
  — "Fire" biopsy gun; side-cutting needle containing specimen is withdrawn into outer cannula.

Tissue Preparation

If an on-site cytopathologist is not present, follow specimen preparation guidelines established by the institution's cytology/pathology departments.

- *Fine needle aspiration*:
  — Smear specimen on glass slides and place slides in 95% ethanol.
  — Specimens can be placed directly into methanol-based preservative solution.
- *Core biopsy*:
  — Place nonfocal biopsy specimens in formalin.
  — Focal biopsy specimens may be placed in sterile saline but this is dependent on institutional pathology department preference.
- *Special circumstances (as guided by clinical history and prior imaging)*:
  — *Lymphoma*: Send separate FNA specimen in sterile saline for flow cytometry.
  — *Breast cancer*: Hormone receptor/Her2 analysis.
  — *Prostate cancer*: PSA stain.
  — *Microbiology*: Gram stain, culture and sensitivity, fungal stain and culture, AFB, TB culture.
  — *Pediatric patients*: Genetic testing depending on tumor type.

Immediate Post-procedure Care

- *Ultrasound-guided biopsy*:
  — After needle removal, scan biopsy site and Morrison's pouch for hemorrhage.
  — Chest radiograph if suspicion for pneumothorax.
- *CT-guided biopsy*
  — Post-procedure scan to assess for hemorrhage, pneumothorax, and hemothorax.
- *Hemorrhage during biopsy*:
  — Earliest sign of clinically significant hemorrhage is tachycardia. Obtain type and cross, consider transfusion, and plan hospital admission.
  — Gelfoam embolization of the needle tract may be performed at the end of the procedure if hemorrhage from hypervascular lesions is encountered during the biopsy.
  — Gelfoam slurry is instilled by syringe through the coaxial needle as the needle is withdrawn.

Follow-up and Post-procedure Medications

- Can consider repeat percutaneous biopsy if specimens are nondiagnostic.
- Surgical biopsy may be required in select cases.
- *Post-procedure pain*:
  — Assess vital signs; new tachycardia raises suspicion for clinically significant hemorrhage.
  — Mild-to-moderate pain is an expected finding; can treat with NSAIDs; rarely requires narcotics

Results

- Accuracy ranges from 83% to 100%.
- Errors in diagnosis are infrequent.
  — False-negative results >>> false-positive results.

Complications

- Complication rates range from 0% to 6%; most studies estimate < 2%.
- Complication rates slightly higher with larger needles.
- Clinically significant hemorrhage < 2%.

- — How to minimize risk:
  - — Correction of coagulation parameters
  - — Needle path avoidance of intrahepatic branch vessels
  - — Minimize number of punctures of liver capsule
  - — Gelfoam embolization of needle tract
- • Pneumothorax:
  - — Asymptomatic patients with small pneumothoraces may have a 2 h follow-up chest radiograph.
  - — If pneumothorax is stable or decreased in size, may discharge patient with instructions to seek medical attention if worsening pain or dyspnea.
  - — Otherwise, consider chest tube placement.
  - — How to minimize risk:
  - — Minimize number of transpleural or transpulmonary needle punctures.
  - — Use subcostal rather than intercostal approach when possible.
- • Bowel injury and infection are rare and may manifest as a delayed complication such as abscess.
- • Tract seeding is exceedingly rare.
- • Mortality $< 0.1\%$.

Key Points

> Review preprocedural imaging to confirm need for biopsy and plan approach to focal lesions.
> Ultrasound is the preferred image-guiding modality.
> CT is used for focal liver biopsy of lesions not well demonstrated on ultrasound.
> Coaxial technique is preferred to minimize number of passes through liver capsule.
> Immediate post-procedure imaging may detect early complications such as hemorrhage or pneumothorax.
> Insufficient material is the most common cause of nondiagnostic biopsy.

Suggested Reading

1. Gazelle GS, Haaga JR. Guided percutaneous biopsy of intraabdominal lesions. *AJR Am J Roentgenol.* 1998;206:429-935.
2. Smith EH. Complications of percutaneous abdominal fine-needle biopsy. *Radiology.* 1991;178:253-258.
3. Charbonneau JW, Reading CC, Welch TJ. CT and sonographically guided needle biopsy: current techniques and new innovations. *AJR Am J Roentgenol.* 1990;154:1-10.
4. Martino CR, Haaga JR, Bryan PJ, LiPuma JP, El Yousef SJ, Alfidi RJ. CT-guided liver biopsies: eight years' experience. *Radiology.* 1984;152:755-757.

Chest Biopsy

Aoife N. Keeling

Clinical Features

- Lung cancer remains the leading cause of cancer death in both males and females alike.
- Both active and passive cigarette smoking result in lung cancer, with other inhaled carcinogens, including radon gas and asbestos, playing a more minor causative role.
- Four histological types of lung cancer: adenocarcinoma (most common), squamous cell carcinoma, large cell carcinoma, and small cell undifferentiated carcinoma.
- Not all lung masses are primary lung cancer, with greater than 70% of multiple lung nodules representing metastatic deposits.
- Early reports of percutaneous transthoracic needle biopsy of the lung were published in the late 1800s and since then needle biopsy has gained wide acceptance for diagnosing malignant and benign lung lesions.

Diagnostic Evaluation

Clinical

- History and examination to rule out any contraindications (see below).

Laboratory

- Full blood count, coagulation screen, respiratory function tests to make sure that the patient could tolerate a pneumothorax.

A.N. Keeling
Department of Interventional Radiology, Guy's and St. Thomas' NHS Trust, London, UK

D.A. Gervais and T. Sabharwal (eds.),
Interventional Radiology Procedures in Biopsy and Drainage,
DOI: 10.1007/978-1-84800-899-1_3, © Springer-Verlag London Limited 2011

Imaging

CXR

- Useful to determine if the lung lesion is visible (fluoroscopic-guided biopsy)
- To determine any contraindications (pneumonectomy/bullae/severe emphysema/pneumothorax)
- To diagnose any postbiopsy complications (pneumothorax)

CT

- Accurate lesion localization, location of fissures, detection of bullae, etc. that may cause problems.

PET

- Useful to confirm diagnosis and detect metastasis

US

- Useful for pleural-based lesions or lesions invading the chest wall

Lung Needle Biopsy Indications

- Solitary or multiple lung lesion/lesions greater than 5 mm in diameter where the histology is unknown and obtaining histology will alter the clinical management of the patient.

Lung Needle Biopsy Contraindications

Absolute

- Patients or family refusing to give consent.
- Coagulopathic with INR > 1.5, APTT > 40, platelets < 70, 000 or receiving full anticoagulation with low molecular heparin.
- Lesion smaller than 5 mm in diameter.

- Cases where a tissue diagnosis will not alter the clinical management plan for the patient.

Relative

- Large bullae (high risk of pneumothorax)
- Previous pneumonectomy/single lung
- Severe emphysema (may not be able to tolerate a pneumothorax)
- Coexisting contralateral pneumothorax

Relevant Anatomy

- Establish the lesion location, peripheral lesions are best suited to percutaneous biopsy, however, central lesions adjacent to the main bronchi are better suited to endoscopic biopsy.
- Establish the location and number of fissures adjacent to the lung lesion or within the pathway of the biopsy needle trajectory. Lung windows on the CT thorax are most valuable.
- Establish the location of adjacent arteries and veins (may need to administer intravenous contrast medium prior to the CT) in order to plan the needle trajectory to avoid these vascular structures.

Aberrant Anatomy

- Accessory fissures: document their presence in order to avoid traversing them with the biopsy needle.
- Pre-procedure imaging should be closely reviewed to document any normal variants, which would interfere with a safe procedure such as dextrocardia, right-sided or double aortic arch.

Patient Preparation

- Ensure an appropriate clinical indication for the lung biopsy exists, i.e., a histological diagnosis is required to guide further clinical management.
- Informed consent, FBC, and INR.

Equipment/Tools

Needle Types

Fine needle/large gauge needle/cutting core biopsy needle.

- Core biopsy avoids the need for a cytopathologist to be in attendance as the tissue core is placed in formalin and sent to the histology laboratory. However, with a fine-needle aspiration biopsy (FNAB), there should be a cytopathologist in attendance to view the slides and ensure that sufficient cells are aspirated.
- Which needle to use? Lesions from 5 mm to 1 cm in diameter would be better suited to FNAB, with lesions > 1 cm suitable for coaxial cutting needle biopsy.
- Coaxial versus Tandem? Coaxial needle use is safer than tandem needle use due to the fact that the pleura is only punctured once with the coaxial technique and an infinite number of biopsies are then possible. With the tandem technique a smaller needle is placed into the lesion and then the biopsy needle is placed in a parallel trajectory into the lesion, necessitating at least two pleural punctures for only one core and more pleural punctures for more cores. The pneumothorax rate increases with more pleural punctures.
- Coaxial needle technique allows for plugging of the needle tract to minimize pneumothorax occurrence and aspiration can be performed if pneumothorax does occur.

Results

- Percutaneous fine-needle aspiration biopsy (FNAB) is a safe technique for diagnosing malignant lung lesions, with a diagnostic accuracy rate of 94% and a sensitivity of 95%, but its diagnostic sensitivity rate in benign lung diseases is reported to be lower than 50% in most series.
- Coaxial automated cutting needle (18–20G) technique has a high diagnostic sensitivity rate for malignant (88–95%) and benign diseases (71–97%). Lesion size (<1.5 cm [technically difficult] and >5 cm [central necrosis]) together with a benign histology negatively affect a correct histological diagnosis following cutting needle biopsy.

Pre-procedure Medication/Sedation/Analgesia

- Local anesthesia, usually 10 mL 1% lignocaine, should be administered into the overlying skin, subcutaneous tissues, chest wall musculature, and the overlying pleural surface.
- Sedoanalgesia. However, some interventionalists do not use sedation to ensure patient cooperation with breath hold during needle insertion and firing.

Procedure

Planning an Access Route

- Needle pathway should be planned on the diagnostic CT prior to intervention. Care should be taken to avoid fissures, bullae, and vessels. The needle trajectory should be pointed away from the heart and great vessels. The needle should be placed above the rib below when traversing the intercostal space to avoid the subcostal neurovascular bundle.
- For subpleural lesions, a longer oblique needle path has been shown to increase diagnostic accuracy and safety, as the guiding needle is less likely to become displaced into the pleural cavity if it has a longer intra parenchymal tract. Thus, pneumothorax rate is reduced and tissue sampling is more accurate.
- Patient should be prone or supine, whichever gives the shorter and safer route to the lesion, as this will be a more stable position and more comfortable for the patient.

Image Guidance

- CT is now the method of choice to guide lung biopsy with both FNAB and coaxial cutting needle techniques. CT allows excellent pre-procedure needle trajectory planning and risk minimization. Needle guidance is accurate, but not usually in real time. Immediate detection of postbiopsy complications is possible with CT, which can also be used to guide chest drain insertion.
- Fluoroscopy was previously commonly used to guide lung needle biopsy for lesions visible on plain x-ray. However, most centers now prefer CT guidance to minimize complications.
- Ultrasound (US) is useful for the biopsy of subpleural lesions where the continuous real-time nature of the imaging is valuable in guiding the needle into the lesion. However, US is of no use in guiding the biopsy of intraparenchymal lung lesions due to the inability of US to penetrate aerated lung.

Performing the Procedure

Technique

- Aseptic technique should be performed with full sterile precautions taken.
- Skin access site is determined and cleaned with appropriate agent and infiltrated with local anesthesia. Small incision is made and the outer guiding 19G coaxial needle is placed into the subcutaneous tissue.
- Needle trajectory is then checked with the imaging modality and adjusted if necessary prior to pleural puncture.

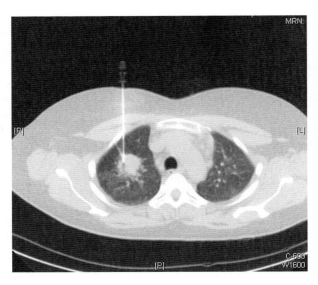

Fig. 1 19G guiding coaxial needle positioned within the lateral portion of an RUL lesion to avoid the medially placed vessels. The 20G cutting needle was then placed via this guiding needle into the lesion to obtain the tissue cores

- A single pleural puncture should be made and the needle path adjusted again as necessary with image localization until the lesion is entered successfully. The outer guiding needle should be positioned on the near edge of the lung lesion (Fig. 1).
- Breath hold should be performed by the patient during needle advancement to limit lung parenchymal injury.
- With the guiding needle in position, the inner stylet is removed, with the operator's finger placed over the lumen to avoid any air aspiration (could cause pneumothorax or air embolism) and the 20G cutting needle is placed into the lesion via the guiding needle.
- A staged firing needle is preferred to minimize vessel injury but yet obtain an adequate tissue core. When fired, the cutting needle is removed, stylet replaced into the needle guide, and the tissue core removed from the cutting needle, inspected and placed into 10% formalin.
- The angle of the guiding needle can be changed manually by steering it under imaging guidance to ensure sampling from a different location within the lesion with subsequent cutting needle biopsy.

End Point

- Most operators obtain at least two tissue cores, however, with the 20G cutting needle the cores tend to fragment, thus if it is felt that not enough tissue is present, there has been no bleeding and the guiding needle is still in place, then another core can be obtained.
- Prior to guiding needle removal imaging is employed to ensure that no pneumothorax has occurred. The guiding needle is then removed slowly to allow the lung parenchyma to recoil around the needle tract to minimize the occurrence of a pneumothorax.

Immediate Post-procedure Care

- Patient is placed on bed rest, supine at 45° with continuous O_2 saturation monitoring and 15 min pulse and blood pressure monitoring in a dedicated recovery unit for 4 h.
- Routine chest x-ray is performed at 4 h by some interventionalists to ensure no pneumothorax, however, some operators will only obtain a chest x-ray if the patient has a clinical deterioration.
- Many interventionalists now perform lung biopsy as a day case procedure allowing discharge home after 4 h if patient is clinically fit, reserving hospital admission for patients with a post-procedure complication.

Follow-up and Post-procedure Medication

- Clinicians and interventionalists should be available in the event of a late complication such as delayed pneumothorax or hemoptysis, with patients being informed of such complications and the importance of returning to the hospital if they should occur after discharge.
- Clinical follow-up should be performed when the biopsy result is available to determine further management.
- Mild oral analgesia may be required for 24–48 h following the biopsy.
- Repeat image-guided biopsy should be performed in the event of inconclusive histology.

Alternative Procedures

- Iatrogenic pneumothorax can make an inaccessible lesion more favorable for biopsy.
- Some interventionalists have plugged the biopsy tract in order to reduce the incidence of pneumothorax.

Complications: How to Avoid and Manage

- *Pneumothorax*: Lesion depth is the single most important factor in predicting pneumothorax, with subpleural lesions less than 2 cm from the pleura most likely to result in a pneumothorax following coaxial biopsy.

Recent pneumothorax rates are lower for coaxial cutting needles (9–19%) than FNAB (26.9%), with a chest drain insertion rate of 0–3% for coaxial cutting needle biopsy versus 9.2% for FNAB.

Avoidance: Cross the minimum number of pleural surfaces, thus avoid crossing a fissure with the biopsy needle. Use a small caliber needle that will allow an adequate tissue core, i.e., 20G. Some reports have advocated plugging the tract to prevent a pneumothorax.

Management: When using a coaxial needle, perform a check CT prior to removal of the coaxial needle, if there is a pneumothorax at this point, withdraw the coaxial needle into the pleural space and aspirate the air. If the patient experiences respiratory compromise, a guide wire can be placed via the coaxial needle and a percutaneous chest drain placed (Fig. 2).

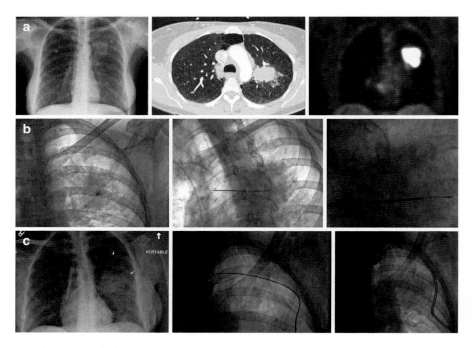

Fig. 2 (**a**) 45 year old female smoker who presented following two episodes of small volume haemoptysis. CXR (left) demonstrates one large spiculated discrete left upper lobe lung lesion. Axial CT thorax (middle) demonstrates a well defined lung parenchymal lesion in the left upper lobe with underlying emphysema and anterior bullous formation. Coronal PET (right) demonstrates an FDG avid left upper lobe lesion. This lesion was scheduled for a fluoroscopic guided needle biopsy. (**b**) Antero-posterior image (left) from the fluoroscopic biopsy procedure demonstrating the 19G guiding co-axial needle positioned within the left upper lobe lesion. Left anterior oblique image (middle) demonstrating the outer 19G guiding needle at the appropriate depth within the lesion. The 20G cutting needle was then advanced into the lesion via the guiding needle (right) to obtain tissue cores. (**c**) Post procedure CXR (left) demonstrates a common post-biopsy complication of a left pneumothorax, requiring fluoroscopic guided chest drain insertion (middle) with subsequent air aspiration and resolution of the pneumothorax (right). Biopsy confirmed adenocarcinoma

- *Bleeding*: Lesion depth is the single most important factor in predicting bleeding, with lesions greater than 2 cm deep most likely to result in parenchymal hemorrhage or hemoptysis following coaxial biopsy. Lesion size ≤ 2 cm is also a predictor in post-cutting needle biopsy hemorrhage as it is felt that there is a higher risk in sampling normal adjacent aerated lung, which will provide no tamponade to bleeding.

Higher bleeding rates with core biopsy (4–10%) than FNAB (2.4–5%), possibly due to the rapid firing of the automated cutting needle, with bleeding being the most common cause of death from a lung biopsy. Thus, certain cutting needles have a staged firing mechanism, i.e., Temno.

  Avoidance: Pre-procedure contrast-enhanced CT to delineate the adjacent vessels and then planning of the biopsy needle trajectory to avoid traversing any large vessels. Avoid sampling any normal adjacent aerated lung parenchyma as this will not offer any tamponade if bleeding does occur. Avoid performing a biopsy if the patient has abnormal coagulation. Avoid a biopsy if the patient has known pulmonary arterial hypertension.

  Management: Most episodes of parenchymal hemorrhage or hemoptysis will settle spontaneously. However, if the patient is hemodynamically unstable, appropriate fluid resuscitation ± blood transfusion is required. Rarely, bronchial or pulmonary arterial transcatheter embolization is required.

- *Infection*: Rarely infection can be introduced into the lung lesion secondary to the biopsy procedure.

  Avoidance: Aseptic technique with full sterile precautions.

  Management: Appropriate antibiotic treatment.

- *Failure:* If insufficient tissue cores are obtained, histology can be inconclusive and thus no diagnosis is made.

  Avoidance: Inspection of the tissue cores at the time of the biopsy procedure to ensure sufficient tissue volume. Use of a coaxial cutting needle system allows multiple cores to be obtained, with just one pleural puncture.

  Management: Repeat the percutaneous biopsy.

- *Air Embolism*: Rare complication due to puncture of a pulmonary vein with air being sucked in and embolizing to the systemic circulation via the left heart, resulting in symptoms resembling those of stroke, transient ischemic attack, seizure, or cardiopulmonary collapse.

  Avoidance: Avoid puncturing a vessel. Place a finger over the outer guidance needle to prevent air being sucked into the needle.

  Management: Remove the biopsy needle. Place the patient in the supine position and administer 100% oxygen. Hyperbaric oxygen therapy is recommended. A diagnosis may be established by performing immediate brain or cardiac CT to search for intravascular air bubbles.

Key Points

> Review all of the pre-procedural imaging to determine that the request for lung biopsy is appropriate, to decide the imaging modality needed to guide the biopsy, to plan the safest needle trajectory, and to determine the appropriate choice of needle system.
> Ensure that the patient is properly prepared for the procedure, i.e., consent, coagulation status, and absence of contraindications.
> If the lesion size permits a coaxial cutting needle system, this is a safe method to obtain high histological sensitivity and specificity rates, and enables a single puncture of the pleura.
> Inspect the tissue cores obtained to ensure adequate samples.
> Perform a check CT following the biopsy to enable early detection of procedure complications.
> Interventional radiologists should be familiar with the potential complications and equipped to manage them prior to chest biopsy performance.

Suggested Reading

1. Pang JA, Tsang V, Hom BL, Metreweli C. Ultrasound-guided tissue-core biopsy of thoracic lesions with Trucut and Surecut needles. *Chest*. 1987;91:823-828.
2. Tanaka J, Sonomura T, Shioyama Y, et al. "Oblique path": the optimal needle path for computed tomography guided biopsy of small subpleural lesions. *Cardiovasc Intervent Radiol*. 1996;19:332-334.
3. Yeow KM, See LC, Lui KW, et al. Risk factors for pneumothorax and bleeding after CT-guided percutaneous coaxial cutting needle biopsy of lung lesions. *J Vasc Interv Radiol*. 2001;12:1305-1312.
4. Yeow KM, Su IH, Pan KT, et al. Risk factors of pneumothorax and bleeding: multivariate analysis of 660 CT-guided coaxial cutting needle lung biopsies. *Chest*. 2004;126(3):748-754.

Mediastinal Biopsy

Alda L. Tam

Clinical Features

- Sixty percent of all mediastinal masses are located in the anterior compartment with the remaining masses originating in either the posterior (25%) or middle compartments (15%).
- The differential diagnosis for a mass in the mediastinum is dependent on the mediastinal compartment from which it arises.
  — Superior: adenopathy, thyroid, cystic hygroma, aneurysm
  — Anterior: thymoma, teratoma/germ cell tumor, thyroid, lymphoma
  — Middle: adenopathy, aneurysm, congential anomaly
  — Posterior: neurogenic tumors, nerve root tumors, lymphoma
- Accurate staging of non-small-cell lung cancer (NSCLC) patients with enlarged mediastinal lymph nodes is essential as those staged as IIIA are eligible for surgical resection while those staged as IIIB are offered nonoperative treatment.

Diagnostic Evaluation

Laboratory

- Check and correct coagulation profile: platelets, PT/INR, PTT.

Imaging

- Review diagnostic contrast-enhanced CT/MRI or PET/CT to:
  — Determine the location of the mediastinal mass
  — Verify that the mass is amenable to percutaneous biopsy

A.L. Tam
Section of Interventional Radiology, Division of Diagnostic Imaging, The University of Texas MD Anderson Cancer Center, Houston, TX, USA

D.A. Gervais and T. Sabharwal (eds.),
Interventional Radiology Procedures in Biopsy and Drainage,
DOI: 10.1007/978-1-84800-899-1_4, © Springer-Verlag London Limited 2011

— Choose the imaging modality to be used to guide the biopsy
— Preplan needle trajectory and evaluate feasibility for direct mediastinal (extrapleural) versus transpulmonary approach
— Preplan patient positioning for biopsy
— Assess for risk of pneumothorax

Indications

- Establish diagnosis of mediastinal mass of unknown etiology
- Determine staging of non-small-cell lung cancer with N2 nodal involvement
- Evaluate for residual or recurrent disease following treatment
- Determine staging for extrathoracic malignancies

Alternative Therapies (Listed in Order of Least to Most Invasive)

- Endoscopic US-guided biopsy (EUS)
- Endobronchial US-guided biopsy (EBUS)
- Transbronchial needle biopsy
- Mediastinoscopy
- Thoracoscopy
- Anterior mediastinotomy (Table 1)

Contraindications (Relative)

- Uncorrectable coagulopathy
- Uncooperative patient
- Intractable cough
- Severe emphysema or contralateral pneumonectomy (if transpulmonary approach planned)

Specific Complications

- Pneumothorax
  — Reported rates range from 10% to 60%.
  — Risk for pneumothorax increases if both visceral pleural layers are transgressed.
  — Can be managed with the placement of a small bore chest tube attached either to Heimlich valve or Pleurovac.
- Hemorrhage

Table 1 Comparison of various techniques for mediastinal biopsy

Technique	Advantages	Disadvantages	Diagnostic yield
EUS-Bx	• Real-time visualization • Access to lower paratracheal, subcarinal and AP window LNs	• Pretracheal and high paratracheal LNs inaccessible due to air artifact from trachea • Core bx not possible	92–97%[a]
EBUS-Bx	• Real-time visualization • Access to lower paratracheal, subcarinal and AP window LNs • Biopsy of endobronchial lesion and adjacent LN possible in same procedure	• Subaortic and paraesophageal LNs inaccessible • Core bx not possible • Wide-spread experience with technique is limited	92–98%[a]
Transbronchial needle biopsy	• Biopsy of endobronchial lesion and adjacent LN possible in same procedure • Best suited for subcarinal or paratracheal LNs • Core biopsy possible	• Inability to visualize needle tip in LN during sampling • Difficult to access other nodal stations	25–81%
Percutaneous needle biopsy	• Access to all regions of the mediastinum • Can be performed under local anesthesia • Core bx possible	• Risk of pneumothorax ranges from 10% to 60%	75–96%
Mediastinoscopy	Gold standard for preoperative staging for NSCLC Access to pretracheal, paratracheal, and anterior subcarinal LNs Direct visualization during biopsy	Requires general anesthesia AP window, retrotracheal, posterior subcarinal, inferior mediastinal LNs inaccessible Complication rate 1–3% including: vascular injury, esophageal perforation, pericardial rupture	83–89%

AP aortopulmonary, *LN* lymph node, *NSCLC* non-small-cell lung cancer, *Bx* biopsy

[a]Diagnostic yield calculated largely from series staging NSCLC. Diagnostic yield dependent on clinical scenario and is lower for lymphoma and benign disease

— Avoid major vessels when planning needle path trajectory to the lesion.
— Mediastinal hematomas are usually self-limited and do not require additional treatment.
— Transgression of pulmonary parenchyma increases risk for pulmonary hemorrhage and hemoptysis.
— Injury to intercostal or internal mammary vessels may result in extrapleural hematoma or hemothorax.

Anatomy

Normal Anatomy

- Assess the lesion and its relationship to critical anatomic structures: major vessels, internal mammary vessels, right and left phrenic nerves, right and left vagus nerves, thoracic duct, esophagus, trachea (see Fig. 1).
- Nodal stations for staging of non-small-cell lung cancer as defined by the American Thoracic Society (see Fig. 2).
- Mediastinal lymph nodes considered abnormal if short axis diameter is >1 cm.

Aberrant Anatomy

- Be aware of anomalous vascular anatomy, which would alter the course and location of major vessels.
- Twenty percent of patients have three internal mammary vessels (two veins and one artery).

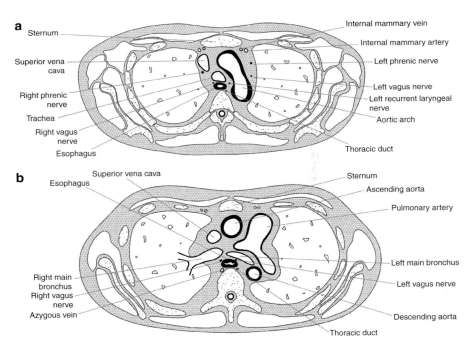

Fig. 1 Cross-section illustration of the location of normal anatomic structures of the mediastinum at the level of the aortic arch (**a**) and carina (**b**)

Equipment

Imaging Modality for Guidance

- CT is the preferred modality for mediastinal biopsy as lesions are often adjacent to major vessels.
  — Non-contrast-enhanced CT is usually adequate for procedure planning if the patient has had previous diagnostic contrast-enhanced CT or MRI.
  — Occasionally, intravenous contrast administration may be necessary to delineate the course of mediastinal vessels and their relationship to the planned needle path or to distinguish vessel from lymph node.
  — Pre-procedural, axial, non-contrast-enhanced axial images are acquired in 3- or 5-mm thick slices to confirm lesion location and plan needle trajectory.

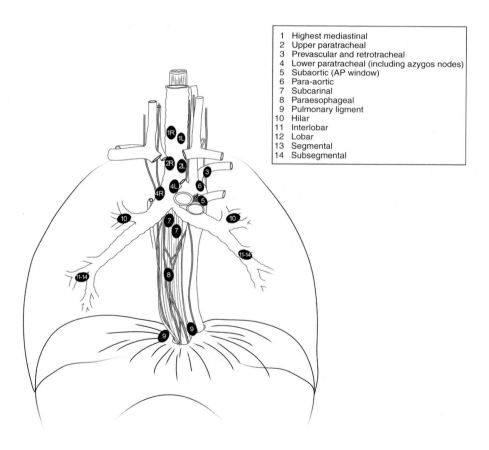

1	Highest mediastinal
2	Upper paratracheal
3	Prevascular and retrotracheal
4	Lower paratracheal (including azygos nodes)
5	Subaortic (AP window)
6	Para-aortic
7	Subcarinal
8	Paraesophageal
9	Pulmonary ligment
10	Hilar
11	Interlobar
12	Lobar
13	Segmental
14	Subsegmental

Fig. 2 Coronal illustration representing the American Thoracic Society nodal stations for staging of non-small-cell lung cancer (NSCLC)

- US is useful for lesions that abut the chest wall and provides continuous real-time visualization of the needle tip in relation to the target lesion and vessels.
  — Preliminary US should be performed to identify the lesion and determine a path for needle biopsy.
  — Transducer selection will depend on the location of the lesion (depth) and either a convex or sector transducer can be used.
  — Color Doppler is helpful for identifying major vessels.

Biopsy Technique

- Single-needle technique: multiple passes are made and a new needle is used each time.
- Tandem technique: small caliber needle is advanced to the lesion under image guidance and subsequent biopsy needles are advanced in parallel to the lesion without image guidance.
- Coaxial technique: a guide needle is placed near or in the lesion to be biopsied and subsequent biopsy needles are advanced through this needle to obtain tissue; technique that is most commonly used for mediastinal biopsy.

Needles

- Small gauge needles provide sample for cytologic evaluation.
  — 20–23G caliber needles are frequently used.
  — Tissue obtained by rapidly moving the needle to-and-fro within the lesion with or without (French technique) suction which is applied using a syringe attached to the needle hub.
- Cutting needles result in extraction of a core of tissue for analysis.
  — 18–20G caliber side-cutting core needles are often used in the mediastinum.
  — Allows for histologic analysis.
- Guide needles should be chosen to accommodate the largest caliber coaxial needle to be inserted.
  — 18–19G thin-wall Chiba needles are common guide needles.
  — A Hawkins needle with an interchangeable blunt/sharp stylet may be particularly useful when the needle path is in close proximity to major vessels, when planning to inject saline for mediastinal widening or when inducing an iatrogenic pneumothorax as the blunt tip should push the visceral pleura away without injury.

Medication

- Mediastinal biopsy is well tolerated:
  — Most can be performed with local anesthesia alone.

— Monitored, conscious sedation using intravenous midazolam and fentanyl citrate can also be used.

— Pre-procedure, prophylactic antibiotics are not routinely recommended.

Biopsy

Patient Position

• Supine, prone, or lateral decubitus positioning will depend on lesion location and planned needle path for biopsy.

Biopsy Approaches to the Mediastinum

1. *Direct mediastinal approaches (extrapleural)*
   (a) *Parasternal approach* (Fig. 3)
      • Position: supine or lateral decubitus.
         — Placing the patient in a lateral decubitus position can move the mediastinum laterally, bringing the mediastinal fat or lesion into contact with the chest wall.
      • Ideal for biopsy of anterior or middle mediastinal lesions, particularly if the lesion or mediastinal fat apposes the chest wall, lateral to the sternum.
      • Needle path should be selected to avoid injury to the mammary vessels.
         — Create "salinoma" by using a 22G needle to inject saline between lateral wall of sternum and internal mammary vessels to allow for extrapleural access to mediastinal mass.
      • Puncture of the brachiocephalic vein and superior vena cava during biopsy of pre- or paratracheal lesions with small caliber needles (22G) has been reported without complication.
      • Normal respiration can alter the degree of apposition between the mediastinum and parasternal chest wall.
         — Can result in transgression of the lung or pleura.
         — Can cause small lesions to move out of the biopsy plane.
   (b) *Paravertebral approach* (Fig. 4)
      • Position: prone or lateral decubitus.
      • Allows access to posterior mediastinal, subcarinal, periesophageal, and paratracheal lesions.
      • Paravertebral path involves passing needle immediately lateral to vertebral body.
         — To avoid intercostal neurovascular bundle, needle should be inserted above the transverse process and over superior edge of rib.
      • Create "salinoma" to widen mediastinum and allow for extrapleural access.
         — Advance 18G blunt tip needle into endothoracic fascia.
         — Inject 10–20 cc of saline to create extrapleural space for needle advancement.

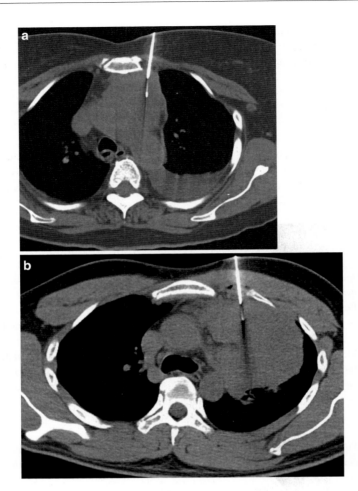

Fig. 3 Parasternal approaches for anterior mediastinal masses in contact with the chest wall. (**a**) Medial parasternal approach: CT scan shows biopsy needle advanced between the lateral wall of the sternum and the internal mammary vessels for biopsy of an anterior mediastinal mass. A 20G core biopsy needle has been advanced through the guide needle for biopsy of the mass. (**b**) Lateral parasternal approach: CT scan shows biopsy needle passing lateral to the internal mammary vessels into the anterior mediastinal mass. A 22G needle has been inserted through the guide needle for biopsy of the mass.

    — Biopsy should be performed promptly because fluid will dissipate.
    — Failure to achieve mediastinal widening indicates that needle is not in the endothoracic fascia.
- Degenerative changes of the spine and orientation of the transverse processes may preclude paravertebral access.
- Potential risk for injury to esophagus, paravertebral vessels, azygos vein, vagus nerves, intercostal vessels, and nerves (including sympathetic ganglia).

(c) *Transsternal approach* (Fig. 5)
- Position: supine.
- Allows access to anterior mediastinal masses that cannot be biopsied safely from a parasternal approach.
  - May occasionally be appropriate access for middle and posterior mediastinal masses.
- Use 18G guide needle to penetrate the sternum by advancing in slow rotating fashion.
  - Local anesthesia should be given at the anterior sternal periosteum prior to needle penetration and again at the posterior sternal cortex to minimize patient discomfort.

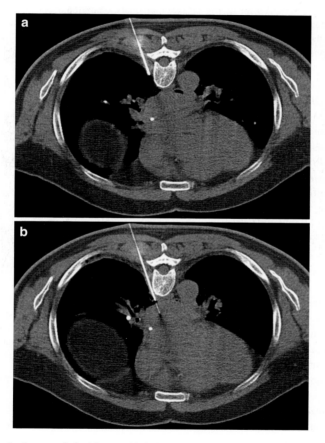

Fig. 4 Paravertebral approach for biopsy of inferior mediastinal mass. (**a**) CT scan shows Hawkins needle advanced to the edge of the paravertebral space. (**b**) CT scan shows that injection of saline resulted in widening of the paravertebral space, allowing for an extrapleural approach to the inferior mediastinal mass. A 22G needle has been advanced through the 18G guide needle for biopsy of the mass.

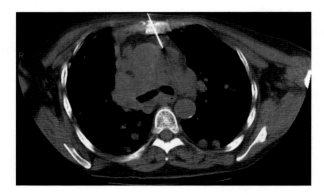

Fig. 5 Transsternal approach for biopsy of aortopulmonary lymph node. CT scan shows biopsy needle advanced through the sternum for biopsy of enlarged lymph node in the aortopulmonary window. The patient has insufficient mediastinal fat to allow for safe access to the lesion via a parasternal approach.

- Needle alignment with the target lesion is particularly important because changes in needle trajectory require total removal of the needle.
- Mediastinal hematomas are occasionally seen following transsternal biopsy, but these tend to be asymptomatic, self-limited, and can be treated conservatively.
- Prior history of sternotomy may make sternal penetration more difficult.

(d) *Suprasternal approach*
- Position: supine with neck hyperextended or semi-erect with head turned to side.
- Provides extrapleural access to masses located above the aortic arch in the superior mediastinum. Also suitable for prevascular, aortopulmonary window and pre- and paratracheal lesions.
- Angulation of the CT gantry may be required to obtain semi-coronal images that will demonstrate the planned needle trajectory from skin to lesion in its entirety.
  - Triangulation may be required to determine angle of needle trajectory when gantry tilt is not used.
- Place US in suprasternal notch and angle caudally to determine avascular path for needle access.
- Major complications are rare with this approach; however, vasovagal reaction may occur.

2. *Transpleural approach*
- Extra-pulmonary access to the mediastinum can be achieved by advancing the needle through an existing pleural effusion or iatrogenic pneumothorax.
- Free-flowing pleural effusions can be redirected into the medial pleural recess, interposed between lung and the mediastinal lesion, with decubitus positioning.
- Induce iatrogenic pneumothorax to create extra-pulmonary access.

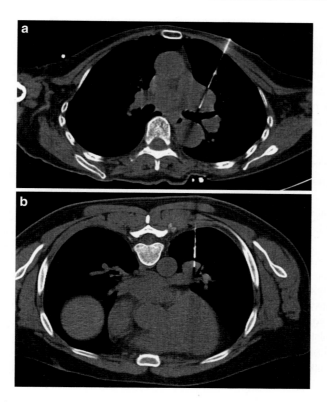

Fig. 6 Transpulmonary approach. CT scan shows biopsy needle traversing the left upper lobe during biopsy of an aortopulmonary window mass (**a**) and left lower lobe during biopsy of a peripheral hilar lesion (**b**).

— Technique should be considered as an alternative to transpulmonary approach in patients with severe emphysema.
— Advance 18G needle to parietal pleura.
— Remove sharp stylet or use a needle with a blunt stylet to advance through the parietal pleura.
— Inject air into pleural space to collapse lung.
— Aspirate out air after biopsy to reexpand the lung.
3. *Transpulmonary approach* (Fig. 6)
  • Should be used when a mediastinal lesion is not amenable to an extrapleural approach and is the most common approach used for hilar lesions (stations 10–14).
  • Position patient to allow for shortest transpulmonary path to lesion.
  • Transgression of both layers of visceral pleura increase the risk for pneumothorax.
    — Pneumothorax rates associated with biopsy of hilar lesions range from 33% to 48% with thoracostomy tube rates ranging from 14% to 32%.

— EUS/EBUS-Bx associated with equivalent sensitivity and accuracy rates but lower complication rates (specifically pneumothorax) when compared with percutaneous needle biopsy of hilar lesions.
— Limited access to peripheral stations (12–14) with EUS/EBUS-Bx.
— Because of lower complication rates, EUS/EBUS-Bx may be a reasonable first-line method for obtaining tissue in central hilar lesions (stations 10–11).

- Avoid major fissures, emphysematous bullae, and major vessels.

Clinical Scenarios

Clinical context and pathological consideration should determine the type of tissue samples obtained.

- Sensitivity of FNA of mediastinal lesion for epithelial carcinoma is 84–100%.
- Diagnostic accuracy is lower for lymphoma, thymoma, germ cell tumor, and neurogenic tumor.
- Core biopsy increases sensitivity for the diagnosis of lymphoma (68% on FNA vs 91% on core biopsy) and is warranted when:
  — Metastatic carcinoma is not the primary working diagnosis.
  — Initial sample from FNA is not diagnostic.
  — Findings suggest benign lesion or noncarcinomatous malignancy.

A negative biopsy of one mediastinal node in the setting of NSCLC does not imply that the mediastinum is cancer-free. The patient may require additional biopsy or mediastinoscopy for complete staging

Aftercare

- Observe patient for 1–3 h to monitor hemodynamic stability and respiratory status.
- For biopsies where a pleural surface was crossed, obtain expiratory chest x-ray immediately and 3 h following procedure to evaluate for pneumothorax.
- Patients with stable, small, asymptomatic pneumothorax may be discharged home.
- Patients requiring chest tube placement can be managed either as outpatients (discharge home with Heimlich valve) or admitted for more aggressive air-leak management (Pleurovac ± suction).

Follow-up

- No special follow-up care is required.

Key Points

> All areas of the mediastinum are potentially accessible with image guidance.
> Extrapleural access to mediastinum is the preferred approach.
> Biopsy technique depends on pathologic considerations.
> Remember tricks of the trade: reposition the patient, create "salinoma."

Safety

> Never start the biopsy procedure until you have personally reviewed the imaging.
> Know the anatomic location of critical structures.
> Be comfortable managing pneumothorax and chest tubes.

Suggested Reading

1. Akamatsu H, Terashima M, Koike T, Takizawa T, Kurita Y. Staging of primary lung cancer by computed tomography-guided percutaneous needle cytology of mediastinal lymph nodes. *Ann Thorac Surg*. 1996 Aug;62(2):352-355.

2. Assaad MW, Pantanowitz L, Otis CN. Diagnostic accuracy of image-guided percutaneous fine needle aspiration biopsy of the mediastinum. *Diagn Cytopathol*. 2007 Nov;35(11): 705-709.

3. Belfiore G, Camera L, Moggio G, Vetrani A, Fraioli G, Salvatore M. Middle mediastinum lesions: preliminary experience with CT-guided fine-needle aspiration biopsy with a suprasternal approach. *Radiology*. 1997 Mar;202(3):870-873.

4. Bressler EL, Kirkham JA. Mediastinal masses: alternative approaches to CT-guided needle biopsy. *Radiology*. 1994 May;191(2):391-396.

5. Caddy G, Conron M, Wright G, Desmond P, Hart D, Chen RY. The accuracy of EUS-FNA in assessing mediastinal lymphadenopathy and staging patients with NSCLC. *Eur Respir J*. 2005 Mar;25(3):410-415.

6. Collins J, Stern E. *Chest Radiology: The Essentials*. Philadelphia, PA: Lippincott Williams & Wilkins; 1999.

7. Detterbeck FC, DeCamp MM Jr, Kohman LJ, Silvestri GA. Lung cancer. Invasive staging: the guidelines. *Chest*. 2003 Jan;123(1 Suppl):167S-175S.

8. Glassberg RM, Sussman SK. Life-threatening hemorrhage due to percutaneous transthoracic intervention: importance of the internal mammary artery. *AJR Am J Roentgenol*. 1990 Jan;154(1):47-49.

9. Glassberg RM, Sussman SK, Glickstein MF. CT anatomy of the internal mammary vessels: importance in planning percutaneous transthoracic procedures. *AJR Am J Roentgenol*. 1990 Aug;155(2):397-400.

10. Goodacre BW, Savage C, Zwischenberger JB, Wittich GR, vanSonnenberg E. Salinoma window technique for mediastinal lymph node biopsy. *Ann Thorac Surg*. 2002 July;74(1): 276-277.

11. Grant TH, Stull MA, Kandallu K, Chambliss JF. Percutaneous needle biopsy of mediastinal masses using a computed tomography-guided extrapleural approach. *J Thorac Imaging*. 1998 Jan;13(1):14-19.

12. Gupta S. Role of image-guided percutaneous needle biopsy in cancer staging. *Semin Roentgenol*. 2006 Apr;41(2):78-90.

13. Gupta S, Gulati M, Rajwanshi A, Gupta D, Suri S. Sonographically guided fine-needle aspiration biopsy of superior mediastinal lesions by the suprasternal route. *AJR Am J Roentgenol*. 1998 Nov;171(5):1303-1306.

14. Gupta S, Seaberg K, Wallace MJ, et al. Imaging-guided percutaneous biopsy of mediastinal lesions: different approaches and anatomic considerations. *Radiographics*. 2005 May–June;25(3):763-786. discussion 86–88.

15. Gupta S, Wallace MJ, Morello FA Jr, Ahrar K, Hicks ME. CT-guided percutaneous needle biopsy of intrathoracic lesions by using the transsternal approach: experience in 37 patients. *Radiology*. 2002 Jan;222(1):57-62.

16. Herth FJ, Eberhardt R, Vilmann P, Krasnik M, Ernst A. Real-time endobronchial ultrasound guided transbronchial needle aspiration for sampling mediastinal lymph nodes. *Thorax*. 2006 Sept;61(9):795-798.

17. Langen HJ, Klose KC, Keulers P, Adam G, Jochims M, Gunther RW. Artificial widening of the mediastinum to gain access for extrapleural biopsy: clinical results. *Radiology*. 1995 Sept;196(3):703-706.

18. Lloyd C, Silvestri GA. Mediastinal staging of non-small-cell lung cancer. *Cancer Control*. 2001 July–Aug;8(4):311-317.

19. Morrissey B, Adams H, Gibbs AR, Crane MD. Percutaneous needle biopsy of the mediastinum: review of 94 procedures. *Thorax*. 1993 June;48(6):632-637.

20. Moulton JS. Artificial extrapleural window for mediastinal biopsy. *J Vasc Interv Radiol*. 1993 Nov–Dec;4(6):825-829.

21. Moulton JS, Moore PT. Coaxial percutaneous biopsy technique with automated biopsy devices: value in improving accuracy and negative predictive value. *Radiology*. 1993 Feb;186(2):515-522.

22. Nakajima T, Yasufuku K, Iyoda A, et al. The evaluation of lymph node metastasis by endobronchial ultrasound-guided transbronchial needle aspiration: crucial for selection of surgical candidates with metastatic lung tumors. *J Thorac Cardiovasc Surg*. 2007 Dec;134(6):1485- 1490.

23. Protopapas Z, Westcott JL. Transthoracic needle biopsy of mediastinal lymph nodes for staging lung and other cancers. *Radiology*. 1996 May;199(2):489-496.

24. Protopapas Z, Westcott JL. Transthoracic hilar and mediastinal biopsy. *J Thorac Imaging*. 1997 Oct;12(4):250-258.

25. Sawhney S, Jain R, Berry M. Tru-Cut biopsy of mediastinal masses guided by real-time sonography. *Clin Radiol*. 1991 July;44(1):16-19.

26. Scalzetti EM. Protective pneumothorax for needle biopsy of mediastinum and pulmonary hilum. *J Thorac Imaging*. 2005 Aug;20(3):214-219.

27. Serna DL, Aryan HE, Chang KJ, Brenner M, Tran LM, Chen JC. An early comparison between endoscopic ultrasound-guided fine-needle aspiration and mediastinoscopy for diagnosis of mediastinal malignancy. *Am Surg*. 1998 Oct;64(10):1014-1018.

28. Shannon JJ, Bude RO, Orens JB, et al. Endobronchial ultrasound-guided needle aspiration of mediastinal adenopathy. *Am J Respir Crit Care Med*. 1996 Apr;153(4 Pt 1):1424-1430.

29. Toloza EM, Harpole L, Detterbeck F, McCrory DC. Invasive staging of non-small cell lung cancer: a review of the current evidence. *Chest*. 2003 Jan;123(1 Suppl):157S-166S.

30. vanSonnenberg E, Casola G, Ho M, et al. Difficult thoracic lesions: CT-guided biopsy experience in 150 cases. *Radiology*. 1988 May;167(2):457-461.

31. vanSonnenberg E, Wittenberg J, Ferrucci JT Jr, Mueller PR, Simeone JF. Triangulation method for percutaneous needle guidance: the angled approach to upper abdominal masses. *AJR Am J Roentgenol*. 1981 Oct;137(4):757-761.

32. Westcott JL. Percutaneous needle aspiration of hilar and mediastinal masses. *Radiology*. 1981 Nov;141(2):323-329.

33. Westcott JL. Transthoracic needle biopsy of the hilum and mediastinum. *J Thorac Imaging*. 1987 Apr;2(2):41-48.

34. Wiersema MJ, Vazquez-Sequeiros E, Wiersema LM. Evaluation of mediastinal lymphade-nopathy with endoscopic US-guided fine-needle aspiration biopsy. *Radiology*. 2001 Apr;219(1):252-257.

35. Williams RA, Haaga JR, Karagiannis E. CT guided paravertebral biopsy of the mediastinum. *J Comput Assist Tomogr*. 1984 June;8(3):575-578.

36. Yasufuku K, Chiyo M, Sekine Y, et al. Real-time endobronchial ultrasound-guided transbron-chial needle aspiration of mediastinal and hilar lymph nodes. *Chest*. 2004 July;126(1): 122- 128.

37. Zwischenberger JB, Savage C, Alpard SK, Anderson CM, Marroquin S, Goodacre BW. Mediastinal transthoracic needle and core lymph node biopsy: should it replace mediastinos-copy? *Chest*. 2002 Apr;121(4):1165-1170.

38. Avritscher R, Krishnamurthy S, Ensor J, Gupta S, Tam A, Madoff DC, Murthy R, Hicks ME, Wallace MJ. Accurracy and sensitivity of computed tomography-guided percutaneous needle biopsy of pulmonary hilar lymph nodes. Cancer 2010; 116:1974-1980.

Bone Biopsy

Farah Irani and Afshin Gangi

Introduction

Bone biopsy is a safe and cost-effective technique, which can be preformed on an outpatient basis under local anesthesia and conscious sedation with minimal complications.

Aim

To obtain sufficient volume of tissue, representative of the underlying disease with minimum risk to the patient.

Indications

1. For pathology:
   (a) Secondary bone tumors/metastasis:
     - Reserved for equivocal lesions on PET CT
     - To determine receptor sensitivity in certain tumors which change therapeutic management; e.g., ER positivity in breast cancer metastasis
   (b) Primary bone tumor:
     - Not performed if complete surgical excision is planned
     - Performed if doubt exists as to the nature of the lesion
2. For bacteriology:
   - For culture and sensitivity to identify the causative organism
   - Determine antibiotic sensitivity

F. Irani(✉)
Department of Diagnostic Radiology, Singapore General Hospital, Singapore

D.A. Gervais and T. Sabharwal (eds.),
Interventional Radiology Procedures in Biopsy and Drainage,
DOI: 10.1007/978-1-84800-899-1_5, © Springer-Verlag London Limited 2011

Contraindications

- Uncorrectable bleeding diatheses
- Inaccessible sites (odontoid process, anterior arch of C1)
- Soft tissue infection with high risk of contamination of underlying bone

Clinical presentation

Tumor	Pain Swelling Pathological fracture
Infection	Fever Swelling Restriction of movement

Pre-procedure laboratory investigations

- Complete blood count.
- INR.

Planning

- Review all diagnostic imaging: CT, MRI, PET CT, bone scan.
- In sarcomas, plan the needle trajectory with the surgeon to ensure excision of the biopsy tract so that tumor seeding and recurrence is avoided. Use coaxial technique. Following biopsy stain tract with methylene blue.

Equipment

1. Semi-automated side notch cutting Temno coaxial biopsy needle (14–18G)
   - For soft tissue and lytic lesions without ossification
2. Ostycut® Bone biopsy needle (14G) (Ostycut®, Angiomed/Bard, Karlsruhe, Germany)
   - For lesions with mild ossification, surrounded by minimal cortex, and spinal biopsies
   - Surgical hammer used for penetration of cortex
3. Trephine needle (Laredo type) (8G)
   - For lesions with mild condensation, primary bone tumors, and lymphoma

Fig. 1 Large osteolytic vertebral lesion biopsied under CT guidance using a 14G Ostycut needle via a transpedicular route. This approach avoids risk of canal transgression and nerve root injury

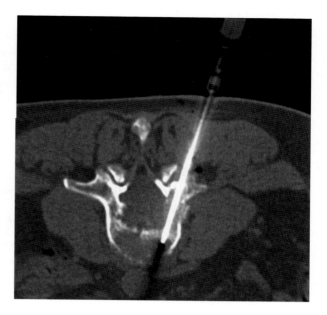

4. Bonopty® Penetration set (14G) (Radi Medical Systems Uppasala, Sweden)
   - For lesions with dense ossification, osteoblastic metastasis, and if dense cortical bone needs to be penetrated (Fig. 1)

Anesthesia

- Local anesthesia and conscious sedation
- Neuroleptanalgesia for painful lesions
- General anesthesia for children

Image Guidance

1. CT:
   - Provides good visualization of bone and surrounding soft tissues
   - Helps avoid damage to adjacent vascular, neurological, and visceral structures
   - Allows for precise needle positioning
2. Fluoroscopy:
   - Offers multiple planes
   - Direct real-time guidance
   - Suffers from poor soft tissue contrast
   - Radiation exposure

3. Combined CT and Fluoroscopy:
   - Recommended for complex procedures especially spine and disc biopsies
   - Fluoroscopy provides real-time needle guidance and intermittent CT scanning allows for accurate needle positioning
   - Performed in a combination fluoroscopy and CT room or by placing a mobile C arm in front of the gantry
4. Ultrasound:
   - Allows real-time guidance
   - For lesions with large soft tissue component and minimal ossification in a superficial location
5. MRI:
   - Used when lesions are not visualized with other modalities
   - In regions adjacent to hardware and implants
   - Intraarticular locations and periarticular cyst aspirations
   - Disadvantages: Not widely available
   - Specialized MR compatible biopsy needle required

Procedure

1. Planning an access route:
   - Planning CT through the region of interest to localize the lesion precisely.
   - Use shortest route from skin to tumor.
   - Route should avoid neural, vascular, and visceral structures.
   - Entry point and needle trajectory plotted on axial CT.
   - Skin entry point marked.
2. Technique
   - After sterile draping, the biopsy trajectory is anesthetized with 1% lidocaine from skin to periosteum using a 22G spinal needle. This needle is then repositioned at the soft tissue tumor interface and a confirmatory scan performed. The biopsy needle is then inserted parallel to the spinal needle using the tandem needle technique. In cases of bone biopsy where cortical perforation is required a surgical hammer may be required to tap the needle into position. Frequent scans are performed to check for correct needle trajectory as once in bone it is very difficult to change direction. The use of fluoroscopy allows for real-time monitoring of needle progression. Once within the lesion, as checked with CT, sampling is performed.
   - For histo-pathological examination the specimen is fixed in 10% formalin. If bacteriological analysis is necessary the specimens are not fixed and sent for culture in normal saline. Single use needles are preferred for biopsies.
   - On completion of biopsy, the needle is removed and compression applied. A check CT through the biopsy site is done to rule out hemorrhage.

Peripheral long bone: The approach has to be orthogonal to the bone cortex, as this avoids the needle tip slipping off the cortex. The approach must avoid tendons as well as nerves, vessels, visceral, and articular structures.

Flat bones (scapula, ribs, sternum, and skull): An oblique approach using a 30–60° angle is recommended. This approach is a compromise between the tangential approach, which avoids damage to underlying structures and the orthogonal approach which avoids slippage of the needle tip.

Pelvic girdle: A posterior approach is used to avoid the sacral canal and nerves.

Vertebral body biopsy: Different approach routes can be selected depending on vertebral level biopsied: the antero-lateral route for the cervical level; the transpedicular or intercostovertebral route for the thoracic level; and the posterolateral or transpedicular route for the lumbar level.

For the vertebral posterior arch a tangential approach is used to avoid damage to underlying neural structures.

Vertebral disc biopsy: As for vertebral biopsies the approach changes depending on the level at which the biopsy is performed. For the lumbar level, a transforaminal route using the "Scotty dog" technique is used to gain access to the disc. At the thoracic level the intercosto-transverse route is used with needle advanced in the direction of the fluoroscopic beam which is directed 35° from the patient's saggittal plane (Fig. 2).

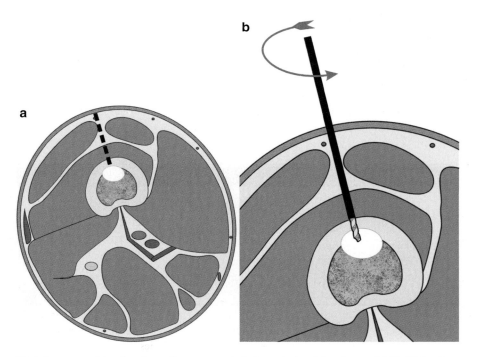

Fig. 2 Image graphics showing safe access route to bony lesion (**a**) and use of drill (**b**) to allow easier penetration of cortex

Post Biopsy Care

- Bed rest for 4 h
- Monitor vitals every 30 min for 4 h
- Pain controlled with oral analgesics

Complications

Incidence: 0–2%

1. Infection: Maintain strict sterility.
   For immunocompromised patients perform under antibiotic cover
2. Hematoma
3. Reflex sympathetic dystrophy
4. Neural and vascular injury
5. Pneumothorax following thoracic biopsy
6. Tumor seeding : Rare but real possibility.
   Plan needle trajectory with consulting surgeon
7. Needle tip breakage within lesion (namely, cortical bone)

Results

Diagnostic accuracy for CT-guided biopsies ranges from 74% to 96%, but is lower for spinal and infectious etiologies.

Key Points

> Carefully review all diagnostic imaging
> Carefully plan needle trajectory
> For sarcomas plan biopsy trajectory with consultant surgeon
> Maintain strict sterility
> Use appropriate needle for appropriate lesion
> Revise anatomy to avoid surrounding important vascular and neural structures

Adrenal Biopsy

David J. Grand and William W. Mayo-Smith

Clinical Features

Incidence

- Adrenal masses have been reported in up to 5% of patients undergoing diagnostic CT,[1] almost always discovered as incidental findings.
- The vast majority of these lesions are adenomas. In one series of 1,049 consecutive adrenal masses, all lesions in patients without a known history of malignancy were benign.[2]

Differential Diagnosis for an Adrenal Mass

1. Adenoma – may be functioning or non-functioning
2. Metastases
3. Myelolipoma
4. Adrenal hemorrhage
5. Pheochromocytoma
6. Adrenocortical carcinoma

Diagnostic Evaluation

Imaging Features

- The vast majority of adrenal lesions can be definitively characterized on imaging studies, obviating the need for biopsy.
- Most adrenal adenomas (approximately 80%) contain intracellular lipid and are therefore low in attenuation on non-contrast CT.

D.J. Grand (✉)
Department of Diagnostic Imaging, Warren Alpert School of Medicine, Brown University, Rhode Island Hospital, Providence, RI, USA

D.A. Gervais and T. Sabharwal (eds.),
Interventional Radiology Procedures in Biopsy and Drainage,
DOI: 10.1007/978-1-84800-899-1_6, © Springer-Verlag London Limited 2011

- An adrenal mass measuring ≤10 HU on non-contrast CT is diagnostic of an adenoma.[3]
- The presence of intracellular lipid also causes adrenal masses to lose signal on chemical shift (out of phase) MR imaging.
- An adrenal mass which is brighter than the spleen on in-phase imaging and darker than the spleen on out-of-phase imaging is an adenoma.[4] These techniques will definitively characterize the majority of adrenal adenomas which are referred to as "lipid-rich."
- Approximately 20% of adrenal adenomas are "lipid-poor," meaning that they contain only a small amount of intracellular lipid. These lesions will measure greater than 10 HU on non-contrast CT and will not lose sufficient signal on MR for definitive characterization.
- These lesions are then most commonly characterized with "wash-out" CT. Non-contrast, enhanced, and delayed images are obtained and lesions which de-enhance by 50% at 15 min delay are adenomas.[5]

Contraindications

- Lesions which are characterized as adenomas by imaging *need not* undergo biopsy.
- Adrenal myelolipomas are benign and contain macroscopic fat which is easily demonstrated on either CT or MR imaging. Myelolipomas *need not* undergo biopsy.
- Pheochromocytomas are often bright on T2-weighted MRI and need not undergo a biopsy as the biopsy may precipitate a hypertensive crisis.
- Pheochromocytoma is diagnosed by serum catecholamine levels or 24-h urinary metanephrine and catecholamine levels.
- Pheochromocytoma may mimic other adrenal lesions such as cyst or adenoma or even myelolipoma on imaging studies, so that any adrenal mass in the setting of elevated metanephrines and catecholamines must be considered pheochromocytoma.[6]

Indications

- Lesions which cannot be characterized by the above methods or are large (>4 cm) and heterogeneous may be referred for adrenal biopsy.

Alternatives

- Masses which are highly suspicious for adrenal cortical carcinoma (isolated adrenal mass >4 cm with central necrosis and/or irregular margins in a patient with no known primary malignancy) should be considered for resection rather than biopsy.

Pre-procedure

- Routine coagulation parameters (INR, platelet count) may be checked prior to adrenal biopsy. Anticoagulants should be discontinued before the biopsy is performed. In otherwise healthy patients without history of abnormal bleeding or use of anticoagulants, some radiologists will not perform these screening hematologic tests.
- All available imaging studies should be reviewed to be certain that the lesion does not have characteristic imaging criteria for an adenoma.
- Evaluate for risk factors for pheochromocytoma and obtain screening plasma catecholamines.
    - Is the patient young and on multiple medications for refractory hypertension?
    - Is the lesion T2-bright?

Relevant Anatomy

- The adrenal glands are in the retroperitoneum, just above the kidneys in the perirenal space and consist of an outer steroid hormone producing cortex and inner catecholamine producing medulla.
- Differentiation of the cortex from the medulla or of the three layers of the cortex is not possible with imaging.
- In cases of congenital ipsilateral solitary kidney or pelvic kidney, adrenal gland remains in the upper retroperitoneum but appears more disc shaped compared to the normal double-limbed appearance on imaging.
- Very rare anatomic variants include adrenal fusion resulting in a single-midline butterfly-shaped gland associated with other congenital midline anomalies.

Procedure Technique

Patient Positioning

- Whenever possible, biopsy an adrenal mass in the decubitus position with the ipsilateral side down (Fig. 1). This technique causes decreased excursion of the dependent diaphragm allowing direct axial in-plane access to most adrenal lesions without transgressing the lung.[7]
- If the lung remains in a projected in-plane axial approach to the adrenal mass, either in prone or decubitus position, an inferior to superior needle trajectory can be performed with either triangulation or gantry angulation.
- Triangulation is based on the Pythagorean theorem calculated based on the right triangle formed by measuring the depth of the target on an axial image and the distance

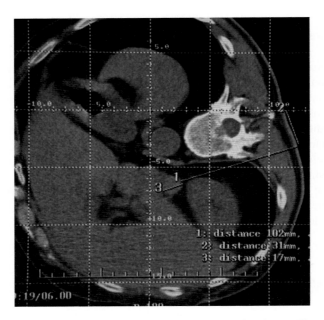

Fig. 1 Pre-procedural CT image in patient with indeterminate right adrenal mass. The patient is in the right lateral decubitus position and the procedure is planned using measurements on the CT console

cephalad from that point of the skin entry site. The needle trajectory distance is the length of the hypotenuse of the right triangle.

- Gantry angulation involves a slight tilt of the gantry to create an oblique axial image allowing the needle to course caudal to cephalad in the oblique axial plane of the image and making imaging of the entire needle possible if it stays in this plane.
- If this is not possible, a direct prone, trans-hepatic, or even an anterior approach may be utilized.[3]

Equipment and Biopsy

- A coaxial needle biopsy device is preferred as it allows the operator to obtain multiple samples without repositioning the outer needle (Fig. 2).
- Generally, 16–19G outer needles are used.
- Placement of the coaxial introducer allows both passage of an aspirating needle (19–22G) for FNA and a core needle (17–20G) for cores.
- Scout CT images are obtained and the skin entry site is marked. Anesthetize the skin and deeper soft tissues with local anesthetic.
- Advance the outer 19G needle of the coaxial system to the adrenal margin.
- Place the20G biopsy needle coaxially through the 19G needle so it extends through the adrenal mass.

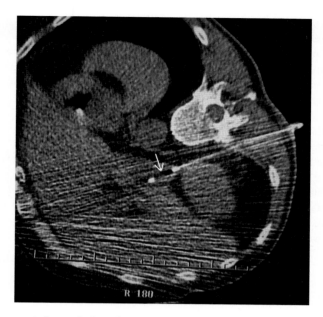

Fig. 2 CT fluoroscopic image during adrenal biopsy in same patient. The inner needle extends to the adrenal mass and the "trough" is deployed through the lesion (*arrow*)

- Obtain at least two passes through the adrenal mass for surgical pathology.
- We observe patients in a holding area for 1 h post procedure.
- Patients do not typically require post-procedural analgesia.
- Discharge instructions are provided and patients are discharged in the care of a guardian. Patients are advised to contact their referring doctor for results of the biopsy in 3 days.

Results and Complications

- Adrenal biopsy has a greater than 90% accuracy, a sensitivity of 81%, and a specificity of 99%.[8]
- The positive predictive value of 99% makes adrenal mass biopsy very useful in staging established extra-adrenal malignancy such as lung cancer.[8]
- The negative predictive value of 80% makes adrenal biopsy less useful to separate benign from malignant conditions.[8]
- Complication rate is under 3%.[8]
- The most common complication is hemorrhage.[8]
- Other potential complications are rare and include pneumothorax, adjacent organ injury (kidney, pancreas, bowel), infection, or hypertensive crisis if an unsuspected pheochromocytoma undergoes biopsy.

Key Points

> Adrenal masses are extremely common and almost always found incidentally on CT examinations performed for another reason.
> The vast majority of adrenal masses are benign adenomas – even in patients with known malignancy.
> Adrenal mass biopsy is indicated in patients with:
> — An indeterminate adrenal mass and a known history of malignancy
> — An indeterminate adrenal mass >4 cm
> For patients with an adrenal mass and no history of malignancy, perform screening plasma catecholamines or 24 h urinary metanephrines and catecholamines *before* biopsy to exclude pheochromocytoma.
> The lateral decubitus position with the ipsilateral (mass-side down) is useful to minimize the incidence of pneumothorax.
> Preferred needle=Coaxial 18–20G biopsy gun.

Suggested Reading

1. Kloos RT, Gross MD, Francis IR, Korobkin M, Shapiro B. Incidentally discovered adrenal masses. *Endocr Rev.* 1995;16:460-484.
2. Song JH, Chaudry FS, Mayo-Smith WW. The incidental adrenal mass on CT: prevalence of adrenal disease in 1, 049 consecutive adrenal masses in patients with no known malignancy. *AJR.* 2008;190:1163-1168.
3. Mayo-Smith WW, Boland GW, Noto RB, Lee MJ. State of the art adrenal imaging. *Radiographics.* 2001;21:995-1012.
4. Outwater EK, Siegelman ES, Radecki PD, Piccoli CW, Mitchell DG. Distinction between benign and malignant adrenal masses: value of T1 weighted chemical-shift MR imaging. *AJR.* 1995;165:579-583.
5. Korobkin M, Brodeur FJ, Francis IR, Quint LE, Dunnick NR, Londy F. CT time–attenuation washout curves of adrenal adenomas and nonadenomas. *AJR.* 1998;170:747-752.
6. Blake MA, Kalra MK, Maher MM, et al. Pheochromocytoma: an imaging chameleon. *Radiographics.* 2004;24:S87-S99.
7. Heiberg E, Wolverson MK. Ipsilateral decubitus position for percutaneous CT-guided adrenal biopsy. *J Comput Assist Tomogr.* 1985;9(1):217-218.
8. Welch TJ, Sheedy PF, Stephens DH, et al. Percutaneous adrenal biopsy: review of a 10-year experience. *Radiology.* 1994;193(2):341-344.

Renal Biopsy

Onofrio A. Catalano and Anthony E. Samir

Clinical Features

- 47–61% of renal cancers are discovered incidentally.
- 20% of solid renal masses of 3–4 cm are benign, 46% of solid renal masses of <1 cm are benign.
- Small renal masses (<3 cm) are very slow growing (1–2 mm/year).
- Renal cell cancer constitutes the most common kidney cancer and accounts for 12,000 deaths/year in the USA.

Indications

- Indications for solid renal mass biopsy continue to evolve. The following are generally accepted:
  - In the settings of known primary extrarenal malignancy, to differentiate metastatic from concurrent primary renal tumor.
  - To establish a diagnosis when infection is thought to be a potential etiology of a focal renal lesion.
  - Prior to tumor ablation, where a specimen will not be available for pathologic evaluation.
  - Borderline surgical candidates, where biopsy may obviate the need for surgery by diagnosing a fat poor angiomyolipoma. The evidence for this approach is strongest for small masses, which have a higher pretest probability of benignity.

O.A. Catalano (✉)
Abdominal and Interventional Radiology Department, Massachusetts General Hospital, Boston, MA, USA and SDN Istituto di Ricerca Diagnostica e Nucleare, Napoli, Italy

D.A. Gervais and T. Sabharwal (eds.),
Interventional Radiology Procedures in Biopsy and Drainage,
DOI: 10.1007/978-1-84800-899-1_7, © Springer-Verlag London Limited 2011

Contraindications

- No absolute contraindications.
- Relative contraindications: coagulopathy, relevant anatomy.

General Principles

Patient Preparation

- *Diet*: Nil by mouth 4–6 h prior to the procedure
- *Consent*: Bleeding, infection, organ, nerve or vascular injury, pseudoaneurysm, and non-diagnostic biopsy (~5%). Bleeding requiring admission or transfusion was reported in 2% of 400 focal renal lesion biopsies at our institution, with no case requiring surgical or endovascular intervention.
- *Coagulation*: It is recommended that INR, PTT, platelets be routinely checked pre-procedure.
- *Antibiotics*: Not routinely administered.
- *Imaging*: A recent intravenous contrast-enhanced CT or MR study of the upper abdomen is preferred, as it facilitates accurate pre-procedural planning. Hypertrophy of a column of Bertin may simulate a focal mass lesion. Dedicated renal imaging by CT or MR is able to distinguish between a mass and this anatomic variant.

Access

- Depending on tumor location and relationship with surrounding structures, renal biopsies may be performed in the prone, supine, lateral decubitus, and oblique positions.
- A posterior approach with the patient in the lateral decubitus position with the side of the lesion dependent is preferred. This approach stabilizes the kidney within the retroperitoneal fat, reduces renal respiratory motion, and reduces bowel and pulmonary interposition. The renal vessels and collecting system are largest in the renal sinus. Consequently, a biopsy trajectory that does not traverse the renal sinus is preferred.

Image Guidance

- Computed tomography (Fig. 1) or real-time ultrasound guidance.
- Contrast medium can be administered if better localization of the tumor is needed.
- Magnetic resonance guidance provides better soft tissue contrast, and may be useful when intravenous contrast cannot be given but is only available in a few centers and is costly owing to the need for MR compatible materials and increased procedure room expense.

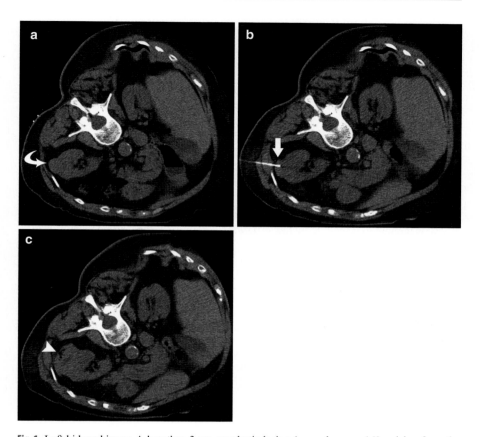

Fig. 1 Left kidney biopsy. A less than 3 cm exophytic lesion (*curved arrow*, **(a)**), arising from the left kidney, was demonstrated on a CT performed for an unrelated indication. The patient was a poor surgical candidate and biopsy was requested. The patient was placed in the left lateral oblique decubitus position and the needle was advanced into the lesion (*arrow*, **(b)**). The post-procedure scan revealed a small amount of expected perirenal hemorrhage and air (*arrowhead*, **(c)**). The biopsy diagnosis was fat poor angiomyolipoma

Sedation-Analgesia

- Conscious sedation can be administered. One percent lidocaine is injected to anesthetize sensitive structures along the planned biopsy path.

Technique

- Multiple fine-needle aspirates and/or core biopsies are obtained.
- In the case of partially cystic lesions, sampling of the solid portion is recommended. The author usually aspirates the cyst fluid and then biopsies the remaining solid portion of the lesion. Water-soluble contrast material may be injected into the cyst to demonstrate mural irregularity and guide biopsy.

General Complications and Management

- In ~2% of the cases, complications, most commonly hemorrhage, may require over-night hospital admission.
- Post-procedure pain may be a manifestation of retroperitoneal bleeding; therefore, a pre-discharge CT scan is obtained in the few patients with more than usual puncture site discomfort.
- Pneumothorax, injury to adjacent organs, and renal colic secondary to obstruction of the collecting system by blood clots may all occur, but are very uncommon.
- It is recommended that all patients be advised to seek medical care if they experience gross hematuria or symptoms of hypotension after discharge. This is exceedingly uncommon.
- Historically there has been concern regarding potential needle track seeding, but the risk is thought to be extremely low (<0.01%).

Tools for Biopsy

Needle Types

- Fine-needle aspiration (FNA): 20–25G needles
- Core biopsy: 15–18G core biopsy needles, placed via a introducer system

Specimen Handling

- FNA specimens are placed in a cytological fixing agent – either on slides or directly into a liquid preservative solution.
- Core biopsies may be placed in saline or formalin depending on local pathology laboratory preference.
- If lymphoma is thought likely, it is recommended that a dedicated aspirate be sent for flow cytometry.

FNA Versus Core

- The diagnostic yield of core biopsy is better than the diagnostic yield of FNA.
- FNA has the theoretical advantage of fewer complications, although this has not been proven in a prospective randomized trial.
- In our experience performing both FNA and core via a coaxial needle system has a higher diagnostic yield than either technique alone and has a low complication rate.

Alternatives

- Imaging surveillance is an alternative for small (≤3 cm) renal masses in older patients, as these lesions grow slowly and have low metastatic potential.

Post-Procedure Care and Follow Up

- Observation for 2 h after biopsy and inspection of the patient's urine prior to discharge is recommended. Bloodstained urine is normal after renal biopsy and generally resolves after several days. Frank hematuria is uncommon. If present, a CT scan is recommended to assess for a hemorrhagic complication.
- Follow up imaging is performed for the majority of tumors which are benign on biopsy.

Key Points

> Renal mass biopsy is a relatively safe procedure that may be performed on an outpatient basis.
> The risk of needle track seeding is extremely low (<0.01%).
> Core biopsy has a higher diagnostic yield than FNA but both together is best.
> Complications are rare <2%.
> The procedure has a high positive predictive value for the diagnosis of renal malignancies, and has been shown to reduce the rate of unnecessary nephrectomy for renal lesions <4 cm in size.
> In the case of benign biopsy histology continued imaging surveillance is recommended.

Other Clinical Scenarios: Non-focal Renal Biopsies

Indications

- Indications for non-focal renal biopsy include diffuse renal parenchymal disease, such as:
  — Renal transplant patients with suspected rejection
  — Patients with suspected glomerulonephritis
  — Patients with renal failure of unknown etiology

Contraindications

- As per focal renal biopsies

Relevant Anatomy

- Glomeruli, which are the main target of diffuse parenchymal diseases, are located within the cortex; therefore, to increase diagnostic yield it is recommended that the biopsy trajectory traverse the cortex in an oblique path, without entering the renal medulla or sinus.

General Principles

Patient Preparation

- As per focal renal biopsies

Access

- In the case of native kidney, a posterior approach with the patient in the lateral decubitus position with the target kidney dependent or a posterior approach with the patient prone are preferred by the authors.
- In the case of a pelvic transplant kidney, a supine position and anterior access are usually preferred.

Image Guidance

- Computed tomography or real-time ultrasound guidance

Sedation-Analgesia

- As per focal renal biopsies

Technique

- Multiple 15–18G core biopsies are obtained.

General Complications and Management

- As per focal renal biopsies

Tools for Biopsy

Needle Types

- Fine-needle aspiration: Not performed
- Core biopsy: 15–18G core biopsy needle

Specimen Handling

- Core biopsies may be placed in saline or formalin depending on local pathology laboratory preference.
- At some institutions a pathologist will review the specimen prior to the end of the procedure to determine that a sufficient number of glomeruli are present in the specimen.

Post-Procedure Care

- As per focal renal biopsies

Key Points

> Non-focal renal biopsy is a relatively safe procedure that may be performed on an outpatient basis
> Posterior approach with US guidance suitable for majority
> Core biopsy needles required

Suggested Reading

1. Wood BJ, Khan MA, McGovern F, Harisinghani M, Hahn PF, Mueller PR. Imaging guided biopsy of renal masses: indications, accuracy and impact on clinical management. *J Urol.* 1999;161:1470-1474.
2. Wunderlich H, Hindermann W, Al Mustafa AM, Reichelt O, Junker K, Schubert J. The accuracy of 250 fine needle biopsies of renal tumors. *J Urol.* 2005;174:44-46.
3. Hunter S, Samir A, Eisner B, et al. Diagnosis of renal lymphoma by percutaneous image guided biopsy: experience with 11 cases. *J Urol.* 2006;176:1952-1956.
4. Uppot RN, Gervais DA, Mueller PR. Interventional uroradiology. *Radiol Clin North Am.* 2008;46:45-64.

Pancreatic Biopsy

Konstantinos Katsanos

Clinical Features

- 28,000 deaths of pancreatic cancer annually in the USA.
- Pancreatic adenocarcinoma is the fourth leading cause of cancer-related death and accounts for 2–3% of all cancers in the USA.
- Majority of adenocarcinomas occur in the head of the gland. Early lymphatic and hematogeneous spread.
- Obstructive jaundice, atypical epigastric and/or back pain, weight loss, cholangitis, and pancreatitis.
- Prognosis is poor with 5-year survival <5%.
- Functioning islet cell tumors present with distinct clinical syndromes (insulinoma with hypoglycemia, gastrinoma with peptic ulcers, glycagonoma with diabetes, VIPoma with watery diarrhea).

Therapy Options

- Surgery (Whipple's pancreaticoduodenectomy), radiation therapy, chemotherapy (5FU, gemcitabine)
- Combinational (surgery and adjuvant chemotherapy and/or radiation)

Laboratory Evaluation

- Evaluate for infection or sepsis, markers specific of islet cell tumors, and blood coagulation parameters

K. Katsanos
Radiology Department, Patras University Hospital, School of Medicine, Patras, Greece

D.A. Gervais and T. Sabharwal (eds.),
Interventional Radiology Procedures in Biopsy and Drainage,
DOI: 10.1007/978-1-84800-899-1_8, © Springer-Verlag London Limited 2011

Imaging

- Ultrasonography, three-phase thin-section CT, gadolinium MR (T1WI and T2WI), multiplanar reformatting of cross-sectional imaging.
- It is crucial that cross-sectional imaging differentiates between resectable (<20%) and unresectable cases (>20%).
- Resectability is defined by freedom of hepatic and lung metastases, regional nodal involvement, encasement of major vessels, and peritoneal carcinomatosis.
- Assess contrast enhancement pattern and discriminate solid from cystic lesions.
- Pancreatic adenocarcinoma presents usually as a hypodense (CT) low signal (MR) mass with associated ductal dilatation.
- Differential enhancement between tumor and normal pancreatic parenchyma is usually maximized 45–60 s post contrast injection (~50 HU).
- Evaluate arterial CT angiographic maps with VRT, MIP, and MPR projections or perform MR angiography and venography.
- If there is no ductal dilatation consider lymphoma, islet cell tumor, cystadenoma, regional lymphnodes, GIST.
- Imaging of ductal system is best performed with ERCP (endoscopic biopsy feasible) and MRCP (plus secretin).
- Beaded dilatation of the pancreatic duct is more frequent with chronic pancreatitis, whereas smooth ductal dilatation is usually a characteristic of carcinoma.
- Ocreotide scintigraphy is useful for the detection of functioning islet cell tumors. Islet cell tumors are hypervascular lesions.
- Metastases to the pancreas may originate from melanoma, renal cell carcinoma, hepatocellular carcinoma, lung cancer, and ovarian cancer.

Indications

- Histological evidence in unresectable patients before palliative chemotherapy and/or radiation
- Exclusion of lymphoma, gastrointestinal stromal tumors, neuroendocrine tumors, metastasis, regional nodal infiltration, or autoimmune pancreatitis
- Differential diagnosis between localized pancreatitis and atypical carcinoma
- Differential diagnosis of cystic mass lesions
- Gene analysis/immunohistochenistry necessary for special monoclonal antibody treatments
- Repeat biopsy if previous is negative and imaging findings are suspicious or atypical

Alternatives

- Endoscopic ultrasound (EUS)-guided biopsy. Permits only fine-needle aspiration (FNA) sampling

Contraindications

Absolute Contraindications

- Non-cooperative patient
- Uncorrectable coagulopathy
- Inability to safely access the lesion/lack of avascular access plane

Relative Contraindications

- Pseudocyst aspiration. Must be followed by drainage
- Splenic or gastric varices if they prohibit safe access
- Older patients with significant co-morbidities who are unfit for palliative therapy

Organ Anatomy

- The pancreas is a 12–15 cm tongue-shaped organ within the anterior pararenal retro-peritoneal compartment.
- It lies anterior to the spine, inferior vena cava (IVC), and aorta and posterior to the left liver lobe, stomach, and lesser sac.
- Pancreatic head, body, and tail extend ventral to the splenic vein (SV).
- Head of the pancreas folds around the confluence of the SV and the superior mesenteric vein (SMV), while the uncinate process extends under the SMV just anteriorly to the IVC.
- The duodenum cradles the pancreatic head in the C-loop.
- Ductal pancreatic system consists of the main pancreatic duct of Wirsung and the accessory pancreatic duct of Santorini draining jointly to the common bile duct and then to the ampulla of Vater. Variant ductal anatomy may be present.

Anesthesia and Sedation

- Adhere strictly to sterility practice
- Anesthetize the whole needle tract with lidocaine 1%
- Intravenous sedation with benzodiazepine/opiate in difficult cases

Image Guidance

- *Transabdominal ultrasound (US)*: US offers real-time monitoring of the needle path as it transverses tissue planes. May be used for bedside biopsy of large pancreatic masses through the gastrocolic ligament.

- *Computed tomography (CT)*: CT has better spatial resolution than US, which is of crucial importance for the targeting of deeply located retroperitoneal organs like the pancreas.
- Angling of the computed tomography scanner gantry may aid accessibility if traditional orthogonal axial views fail to show a safe route of access.
- CT fluoroscopy is an emerging adjunctive tool for high-precision real-time guided targeting of subtle lesions. Scanning parameters must be carefully adjusted to minimize radiation exposure.

Access

- After careful review of the pre-procedure contrast-enhanced CT scan choose the shortest possible needle path. The patient is placed comfortably in the prone or supine or infrequently in an oblique position on the basis of the planned access route.
- Traditional percutaneous access to the pancreas may be intraperitoneal (through the gastrocolic or gastrosplenic ligaments) or retroperitoneal (paravertebral route or through the right or left anterior pararenal spaces toward the pancreatic head and tail, respectively).
- Less commonly, transversal of the liver (avoid the gallbladder, dilated ducts, and the porta hepatis), the stomach (avoid the major mesenteric vessels), the duodenum, rarely the IVC, or renal vein may be attempted.
- In case of transcaval or transvenous puncture avoid co-axial systems and large-bore cutting needles.
- Avoid transgression of the diaphragm, the spleen, small bowel, or the colon.
- Be careful of the superior and inferior epigastric and internal mammary arteries in case of anterior intraperitoneal access (Fig. 1).

Needles and Tissue Sampling

- Goal is to provide adequate tissue samples with minimal complications.
- 18–22G fine-needle aspiration (FNA) or core biopsy needle (CBN).
- Co-axial needle systems are preferred for multiple specimen collection or combination of FNA cytology and CBN histology from the same access.
- During aspiration or needle firing make sure that the tip of the needle is away from major arteries and veins.
- In case of FNA sampling apply forceful back and forth (piston-like) needle movements (>3–5) while aspirating. Remove needle under constant negative pressure.
- CBN better for benign disease, lymphoma, neuroendocrine tumors, and chronic pancreatitis.
- CT-guided pancreatic biopsy has high specificity and accuracy (both ~90%), equivalent to EUS-guided biopsy.

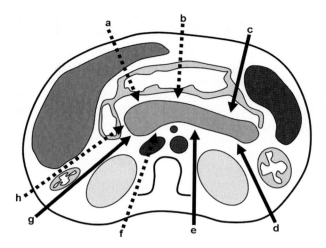

Fig. 1 This figure illustrates common (*black arrows*) and uncommon (*dotted black arrows*) needle pathways to the pancreas including the (**a**) transhepatic (**b**) transgastric (**c**) through the gastrocolic or gastrosplenic ligaments (**d**) from the left anterior pararenal space (**e**) paravertebral (**f**) transcaval or transvenous (**g**) from the right anterior pararenal space, and (**h**) the transduodenal approach (Modified from Maher et al.4)

- On site cytopathologist surely reduces the rate of inadequate specimens.
- Desmoplastic reaction, fibrosis, and inflammation around pancreatic tumors may contribute to sampling error.

Complications

- Local hematoma. Bleeding or hemorrhage is usually self-limited.
- Post-biopsy acute pancreatitis (<1%). Routine supportive care applied.
- Abscess formation, bowel perforation, peritonitis, sepsis, and fistula formation.
- Cystic lesions have a higher risk of superinfection compared to solid lesions.
- Skin or peritoneal malignant tract seeding (<0.1%).
- Total complication rate 1–8%.

Aftercare and Follow-Up

- NSAIDs for analgesia and pain management
- Monitoring of vital signs after the procedure
- Routine blood biochemistry tests the following day

Key Points

> Careful review of pre-procedure cross-sectional imaging to select the safest route of access.
> Access may be intraperitoneal (through the gastrocolic or gastrosplenic ligaments) or retroperitoneal (paravertebral or anterior pararenal spaces).
> Less commonly transgression of the liver, the upper gastrointestinal tract, or rarely the transcaval approach may be attempted.
> Prefer FNA and/or CBN through a co-axial needle system.
> FNA is suggested for carcinoma and risky lesions, whereas CBN for benign lesions, lymphoma, metastases, neuroendocrine tumors, and chronic pancreatitis.

Suggested Reading

1. Lohr JM, Kloppel G. Indications for pancreatic biopsy. Uncommon, but increasingly more important. *Pathologe*. 2005;26:67-72.
2. Amin Z, Theis B, Russel RCG, House C, Novelli M, Lees WR. Diagnosing pancreatic cancer: the role of percutaneous biopsy and CT. *Clin Radiol*. 2006;61:996-1002.
3. Sofocleous CT, Schubert J, Brown KT, Brody LA, Covey AM, Getrajdman GI. CT-guided transvenous or transcaval needle biopsy of pancreatic and peripancreatic lesions. *J Vasc Interv Radiol*. 2004;15:1099-1104.
4. Maher MM, Gervais DA, Kalra MK, et al. The inaccessible or undrainable abscess: how to drain it. *Radiographics*. 2004;24:717-735.

Lymph Node Biopsy

Bradley B. Pua and Stephen B. Solomon

Clinical Features

- Utilized for tissue characterization in:
  - Establishing initial tissue diagnosis
  - Confirmation of metastatic disease which can guide therapy, staging, or prognostication
  - Detecting residual or recurrent disease
- Evaluation for non-tumor etiologies, such as infection or inflammation

Diagnostic Evaluation

Discontinuation of Anticoagulants

In the era of coronary and peripheral vascular stents as well as atherosclerotic disease, more and more patients are presenting to the interventionalist on some type of antiplatelet or anticoagulant.

While there is scattered literature suggesting general guidelines for managing these patients, discussion with the referring physician as to the risk and benefits of temporarily discontinuing these drugs is prudent. For example, the risk of stent thrombosis in a patient discontinuing plavix with a recently placed drug eluting coronary stent may outweigh information garnered from a biopsy.

Most of these guidelines are extrapolated from surgical literature and femoral catheterization and may not apply to the specific biopsy being performed. For instance, biopsy of regions where direct manual pressure cannot be held to achieve hemostasis may require stricter guidelines than biopsy of areas where direct pressure can be held.

B.B. Pua (✉)
Radiology Department, Memorial Sloan-Kettering Cancer Center, New York, NY, USA

D.A. Gervais and T. Sabharwal (eds.),
Interventional Radiology Procedures in Biopsy and Drainage,
DOI: 10.1007/978-1-84800-899-1_9, © Springer-Verlag London Limited 2011

Indications

While there are only a few contraindications for biopsy, it is important to understand the clinical question being answered by the biopsy. Often, the interventionalist can guide which lymph node or organ to biopsy or even the need for biopsy.

Specific Complications

- Biopsy tract seeding is a rare but reported complication, which some authors suggest may be decreased with a coaxial technique. Most of this literature stems from biopsy of HCC with reported rates of 0.6–5.1% utilizing various biopsy techniques. A 0% tract seeding rate utilizing coaxial technique was found in one study looking at 1,012 biopsies.[3]
- Infection, bleeding, and adjacent organ damage. Specific complications are related to access trajectory and proximity to vital structures. Proper patient counseling is imperative.

Anatomy-Specific Considerations

- Abdominal lymph nodes (LN):
  - While abdominal LN biopsies can be performed utilizing multiple modalities (ultrasound, CT, CT fluoroscopy, MRI), sonographically guided biopsies often confer the advantage of the ability to compress the region, decreasing region of transgression, and motion of the targeted lymph node (Fig. 1).
  - While bowel should be avoided, transgression with a small caliber needle is considered safe.
    - Colonic transgression is ideally avoided in immunocompromised patients.
  - Consider endoscopic ultrasound for certain peripancreatic LN or paratracheal LN.
  - Contrast opacification of visceral parenchyma and vessels can help localization of target LN.
  - Adjunct techniques such as saline or air injection to clear biopsy tract can be helpful.
  - While venous puncture is ideally avoided, there are reports of safe transgression of low-pressure veins as well as transgression of the inferior vena cava with small gauge needles.

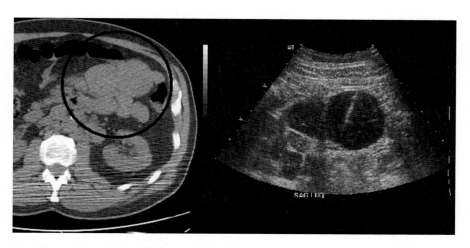

Fig. 1 *From Left to Right*: CT demonstrating bulky mesenteric adenopathy (*encircled*). Lymph node of interest was found to be mobile and was subsequently biopsied under ultrasound guidance, which allowed the operator to use compression to decrease mobility

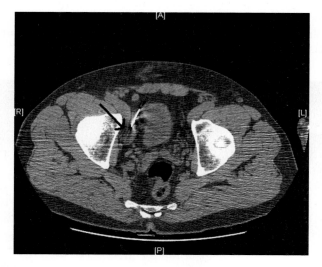

Fig. 2 CT demonstrating biopsy of a lymph node along the deep pelvic sidewall (*arrow*). Unfortunately an approach through the rectus abdominus provided the safest trajectory

- Pelvic lymph nodes:
  - An anterior transabdominal approach is often limited; however, an anterior-lateral approach through the iliopsoas provides access to the external and internal iliac lymph nodes (Fig. 2).
  - For lymph nodes in the presacral or perirectal region, a transgluteal approach through the greater sciatic foramen is often utilized. Needle tract should be

close to the sacrum to avoid the neurovascular bundle traversing the greater sciatic foramen.

— Transosseous or transluminal (transvaginal/transrectal) approaches can also be utilized.

- Paraspinal lymph nodes:
  — CT is often the most useful as osseous structures limit sonographic visibility.
  — Anterior approach for visceral or carotid space lymph nodes.
  — Posteriorlateral approach most common for prevertebral and paraspinal lymph nodes.
  — Lymph nodes anterior to the C1 or C2 vertebrae can be biopsied via a transoral approach, through the retropharyngeal space. This method requires general anesthesia and antibiotic prophylaxis.
  — Contrast injection is useful to identify vascular structures.
- Head & neck lymph nodes – CT and/or MRI is the modality of choice:
  — Subzygomatic approach – allows access to lymph nodes in the parapharyngeal, retropharyngeal, prevertebral, and masticator space (Fig. 3).
    — The needle is inserted in the subzygomatic region laterally, between the coronoid process anteriorly and mandibular condyle posteriorly.
    — Risk of major injury is low; however, there is a theoretical risk of injury to the branches of the trigeminal nerve, internal maxillary artery, middle meningeal artery, and pterygoid venous plexus.

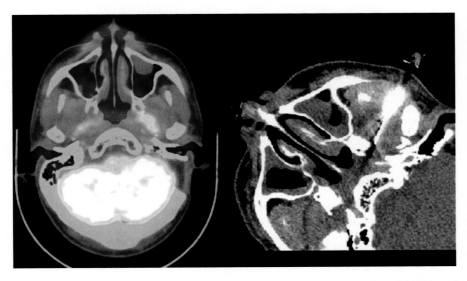

Fig. 3 *From left to right*: Fusion PET/CT demonstrating FDG uptake in the region of the bilateral medial pterygoid muscles in a patient with history of non-Hodgkin's lymphoma. CT demonstrating biopsy needle through the masticator space between the mandibular condyle and coronoid process

— Retromandibular approach – allows access to the inferior portion of the retropharyngeal space, deep parotid space, and parapharyngeal space.
  — Needle is inserted laterally through the parotid gland.
  — Needle insertion and approach anterior to the styloid process helps to avoid the internal carotid artery.
  — Risk of injury to internal and external carotid arteries, retromandibular vein, and the facial nerve.
— Paramaxillary approach – Allows access to the masticator space, carotid sheath, deep parotid space, posterior portions of the parapharyngeal and pharyngeal mucosal spaces, as well as the lateral aspect of the retropharyngeal space.
  — Needle is inserted through the buccal space and aimed posteriorly between the maxilla and mandible.
  — Risk of injury to facial artery.
— Retroparotid approach – allows access to the carotid sheath.
  — Needle is inserted inferior to the mastoid tip and posterior to the parotid gland through the sternocleidomastoid muscle.

Equipment

Needles

- Beveled/angled aspiration needles – generally 20–23G, thin walled with beveled tip
  — Specimens suitable for cytologic examination
  — Examples include Chiba, Turner, and Franseen (Cook Medical, Bloomington, IN)
- Cutting/core needles – generally 18–20G
  — Two main types – side and end cutting

Procedure

Techniques

- Single needle – a new needle is usually used for each successive biopsy pass, requiring guidance for each pass.
  — Disadvantages:
    — Multiple punctures – may result in longer procedure times and increased complications.
    — Potential for increased risk of radiation if CT or fluoroscopy is used.

- Tandem technique – small gauge needle used for localization under image guidance. Subsequently, biopsy needles are advanced in parallel at the same depth, with or without image guidance.
  - Disadvantages:
    - Imprecise localization of biopsy needle tip
    - Multiple punctures
- Coaxial technique – thin-walled guide needle (caliber larger than biopsy needles, typically 17–19G) is advanced under image guidance to in or around lesion of interest. Biopsy needle is passed within this guide needle coaxially to obtain specimens.
  - One puncture.
  - Often preferred for difficult to access areas.
  - Disadvantage: subsequent biopsy passes tend to follow the same path which may yield little additional useful tissue. Side exiting guide needles are available to aid in potentially sampling different parts of the lesion/lymph node.
- Modified coaxial technique – A small gauge needle (23G) with detachable hub is advanced into the lesion. The hub is subsequently removed and and a 19G needle is passed over the 23G into the lesion. The 23G is removed and biopsy samples are obtained with additional needles utilizing the 19G as a guide.
  - Similar advantages and disadvantages as the coaxial technique.

Modality

- Ultrasound – preferred. Advantages include:
  - Shorter procedure time.
  - Allows needle visualization throughout.
  - Biopsy can be performed in single breath hold.
  - Mobile lymph nodes can be compressed fixing them for the biopsy.
  - No ionizing radiation.
  - Equipment is mobile.
  - Real-time post-biopsy imaging.
- CT
  - Not operator dependent
- MRI – not usually utilized secondary to cost and current limits with technology and widespread availability.
  - Multiplanar imaging can be helpful for biopsy in the head and neck regions.

FNA Versus Core

- Decision is often based on comfort of the interventional radiologist at performing biopsy as well as the pathologist/cytopathologist interpreting biopsy specimens.
- FNA utilized when use of large bore needles confers unacceptably high risk (bowel transgression, target structure in close proximity to vital structure, etc.)

- Onsite cytopathologist is associated with increased diagnostic accuracy and cost-effectiveness for FNA.
- FNA confers a poor negative predictive value if cytologic results are negative.
- FNA is often inadequate for subtyping carcinomas and lymphomas.
  - Role of FNA is controversial in lymphoma
    - Core is preferred for initial diagnosis.
    - FNA is considered adequate for post-treatment staging and detection of recurrent or residual disease.

Key Points

> Shortest path between skin and target lesion preferred.
> Injection of saline or air to displace intervening structures in biopsy route can create a more direct and safe path to target lesion.
> Compression with ultrasound can often cut the depth in half, shortening needle path.
> Compression can often mask intervening bowel loops; however, transgression of bowel loops with a small gauge needle is considered fairly safe.

Suggested Reading

1. Winter TC, Lee FT, Hinshaw JL. Ultrasound-guided biopsies in the abdomen and pelvis. *Ultrasound Q*. 2008;24(1):45-68.
2. Gupta S, Madoff DC. Percutaneous needle biopsy in cancer diagnosis and staging. *Tech Vasc Interventional Rad*. 2007;10:88-101.
3. Matmen KE, Nghiem HV, Marrero JA, et al. Lack of tumor seeding of hepatocellular carcinoma after percutaneous needle biopsy after coaxial cutting needle technique. *AJR*. 2006;187:1184-1187.

Splenic Biopsy

Bradley B. Pua and Stephen B. Solomon

Clinical Features

- In oncologic patients, most splenic lesions are metastasis or infectious in etiology.
- Metastasis to the spleen is rare (seen in only 3% of patients at autopsy).
- Splenic biopsy is most commonly used to aid in diagnosis of suspected lymphoma (Fig. 1).
  - Forty percent of patients with known lymphoma have splenic involvement.

Diagnostic Evaluation

Laboratory

- INR below 1.5 recommended
- Platelet count above 50,000/mL (considered low risk of spontaneous hemorrhage as suggested by the College of American Pathologists)

Discontinuation of Anticoagulants

Strongly recommended.

Imaging: It is imperative to have a diagnostic study done prior to the biopsy. The operator then must decide on the imaging modality (i.e., CT, US, or MRI) for the procedure (Fig. 2).

B.B. Pua (✉)
Radiology Department, Memorial Sloan-Kettering Cancer Center, New York, NY, USA

D.A. Gervais and T. Sabharwal (eds.),
Interventional Radiology Procedures in Biopsy and Drainage,
DOI: 10.1007/978-1-84800-899-1_10, © Springer-Verlag London Limited 2011

Fig. 1 Contrast enhanced CT demonstrating a subtle low density lesion corresponding to the lesion of interest (*arrow*)

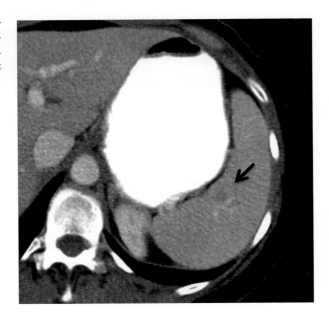

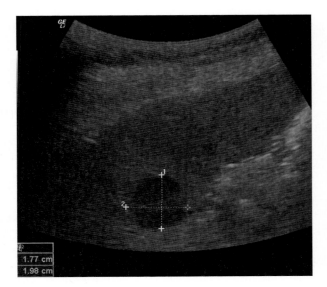

Fig. 2 Ultrasound of the spleen demonstrates a hypoechoic parenchymal lesion in a patient with history of lymphoma

- Plan trajectory to:
  - Traverse the *least* amount of splenic parenchyma, i.e., biopsy peripheral lesions over deeper lesions. Some consider splenic hilar lesions to be contraindicated.
  - Be aware of surrounding structures such as pleura and splenic flexure of the colon.

Indications

- Exclude metastasis.
- Primary diagnosis of lymphoma where the spleen is the only or main organ involved.
- Biopsy may be performed in patients with known lymphoma where new splenic lesions are detected to exclude residual disease, transformation to higher grade, necrosis, or infection.
- Exclude infection in the setting of an immunocompromised patient.

Specific Complications

- Bleeding – most common, 0–5%
  — Usually no intervention is required.
- Pneumothorax is rare.

Anatomy

- Almost entirely surrounded by peritoneum, held in position by the phrenicolienal and gastrolienal ligaments. The lower end is supported by the phrenicocolic ligament.
- Size and weight of spleen is variable dependent on age. In the adult, it usually measures 12 cm in length and weighs about 200 g.
- The splenic artery is a branch of the celiac artery and courses posterior-superior to the pancreas accompanied by its vein. Major branches of the splenic artery include the short gastrics, left gastroepiploic, and pancreatico-magna arteries.
- Supernumerary spleens can be seen in up to 16% of patients undergoing CT.

Equipment

Needles

- 18–22G cutting needles.
  — One study has demonstrated that with a 20–22G coring needles, samples with immunohistochemical staining revealed a diagnosis 85% of the time and 65% of samples had enough tissue to undergo further subtyping.[1]
  — A more recent study demonstrated that 18G has higher diagnostic rate with comparable complication rates when compared to 21G needles.[2]

- 18G cores are often obtained if lymphoma is of diagnostic concern, otherwise FNA with smaller gauge needle often sufficient. It may be worthwhile to discuss this with the primary team and pathologist.

Medications

- Local anesthesia of choice: lidocaine, marcaine, etc.
- Conscious sedation may be utilized if needed.
- Postprocedure pain control is often not required; however, over the counter pain control may be used. Pain that is out of the ordinary should prompt immediate CT to assess for intraabdominal complications.

*Some Interventional Radiologists routinely embolize the biopsy tract with hemostatic material (such as collagen/thrombin).

Procedure

Access

- Plan accordingly after review of the preprocedural imaging
- Traverse minimal to no splenic parenchyma
- Puncture below the12th rib posteriorly or 10th rib laterally to avoid the pleura when possible (Fig. 3)
- Biopsy under suspended respiration if possible
- Biopsy the periphery of the lesion to avoid obtaining necrotic material which may be at the center

Modality

- Ultrasound – preferred
  - Advantages include:
    - Shorter procedure time.
    - Allows needle visualization throughout.
    - Biopsy can be performed in single breath hold.
    - No ionizing radiation.
    - Equipment is mobile.
    - Real-time postbiopsy imaging.
  - Freehand technique or use of biopsy guide may be utilized, although freehand technique allows for more flexibility.
- CT – not operator dependent
  - Usually performed without intravenous contrast unless lesion cannot be localized.

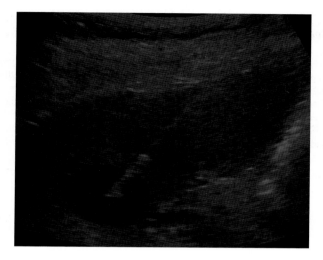

Fig. 3 Ultrasound guided fine needle aspiration demonstrating the needle tip within the lesion of interest

- — Immediate postbiopsy noncontrast CT is obtained to exclude potential complications.
- MRI – not usually utilized secondary to cost, currents limits with technology and widespread availability.

Aftercare

- Bedrest and postprocedure observation for 2–4 h in a monitored setting
- Analgesics not usually required

Followup

- No routine clinic followup; however, phone call from nurse practitioner, nurse, or physician the day after the procedure to assess for delayed complications is suggested.

Key Points

- › The spleen is a highly vascular organ.
- › Biopsy the periphery of a lesion to avoid necrotic centers which are frequent in splenic lesions.
- › Clinical suspicion, in discussion with the referring physician and pathologist, should guide the choice between FNA and core biopsy.

Suggested Reading

1. Lieberman S, Libson E, Maly B, Lebensart P, Ben-Yehuda D, Bloom AI. Imaging-guided percutaneous splenic biopsy using a 20- or 22-gauge cutting-edge core biopsy needle for the diagnosis of malignant lymphoma. *Am J Roentgenol.* 2003;181(4):1025-1027.
2. Liang P, Gao Y, Wang Y, et al. US-guided percutaneous needle biopsy of the spleen using 18-gauge versus 21 gauge needles. *J Clin Ultrasound.* 2007;35(9):477-482.
3. Lieberman S, Libson E, Sella T, Lebensart P, Sosna J. Percutaneous image-guided spenic procedures: update on indications, technique, complications, and outcomes. *Semin Ultrasound CT MRI.* 2007;28:57-63.

Thyroid Biopsy

Anthony E. Samir

Clinical Features

- Sonographically visible thyroid nodules are present in up to 40% of the general population.
- Palpable thyroid nodules and thyroid nodules discovered incidentally on imaging studies have a similar (~10%) risk of malignancy.
- Patients with multiple nodules have a cumulative thyroid cancer risk of ~10%. Nodule multiplicity does not reduce the overall risk of thyroid cancer. One-third of cancers in a multinodular thyroid will be in a non-dominant nodule.

Indications

- Criteria for thyroid nodule biopsy have not been clearly defined. The following are used by the author:
  — Size > 10 mm with microcalcifications.
  — Size > 15 mm and predominantly solid or with coarse calcifications.
  — Size > 20 mm and mixed solid and cystic.
  — AP diameter longer than transverse diameter.
  — Growth – there is no consensus on the definition of nodule growth. At present this assessment is primarily subjective. When available cine-loop data are useful for side-by-side nodule-size comparison.
  — Intranodular vascularity.
  — Any FDG avid thyroid nodule.
  — Any sestamibi avid thyroid nodule.

A.E. Samir
Abdominal Imaging and Intervention Department, Massachusetts General Hospital, Boston, MA, USA

D.A. Gervais and T. Sabharwal (eds.),
Interventional Radiology Procedures in Biopsy and Drainage,
DOI: 10.1007/978-1-84800-899-1_11, © Springer-Verlag London Limited 2011

Contraindications

- No absolute contraindications

Relevant Anatomy

- The thyroid gland is in close proximity to the airway and the laryngeal nerves. Fine-needle aspiration (FNA) may lead to coughing if the laryngopharynx is manipulated, and lidocaine administration may result in transient hoarseness.
- The pyramidal process may project superiorly from the isthmus and should not be confused with a thyroid nodule.

General Principles

Patient Preparation

- *Diet*: Patients do not need to be kept NPO other than in the uncommon circumstance where intravenous sedatives are to be administered.
- *Consent*: Major bleeding, nerve or vascular injury. The risk of permanent hoarseness or voice change is very low ~1/10,000. The risk of major bleeding is extremely low. There is an approximately 10% non-diagnostic rate for thyroid nodule fine-needle aspiration and a 5% false-negative rate for the detection of malignancy.
- *Coagulation*: Not a routinely checked pre-procedure unless the patient takes anticoagulants or has a known coagulopathy. Thyroid FNA safety in patients who are therapeutically anticoagulated with Coumadin or heparin is controversial. Many practitioners perform FNA in this situation without reversing anticoagulation. A platelet count exceeding 50,000 and INR < 1.5 for thyroid core biopsies.
- *Antibiotics*: Not indicated.
- *Imaging*: All patients should have pre-procedural imaging of the thyroid gland and cervical lymph nodes, preferably with ultrasound in the 6 months prior to the procedure.

Access

- The skin of the midline of the neck is usually more pain sensitive; therefore, an anterolateral neck puncture is preferred.

Image Guidance

- Real-time ultrasound guidance with a high-resolution (10–14 MHz) ultrasound transducer

Sedo-analgesia

- One percent lidocaine is injected subcutaneously, followed by 1% lidocaine injected up to the thyroid capsule along the planned biopsy path.
- The thyroid parenchyma is not pain sensitive and therefore should not be anesthetized.
- Mildly anxious patients may be premedicated with an oral benzodiazepine.
- Intravenous sedation is generally unnecessary. Occasionally, very anxious patients may require intravenous sedation with midazolam.

Technique

- Four to six fine-needle aspirates are a reasonable number to perform.
- FNA without aspiration has been shown to be as diagnostic as FNA with aspiration. A reasonable approach is to perform both aspiration and non-aspiration needle passes, and to visually estimate specimen adequacy. If non-aspiration technique yields little macroscopically visible specimen, then aspiration technique can be favoured. If aspiration technique yields specimens that appear macroscopically to contain a large amount of blood, then non-aspiration can be favoured.
- Cystic nodules can be aspirated to completion, with the aspirated fluid sent for cytological assessment and then the collapsed cyst remnant can be sampled (Fig. 1a and b).

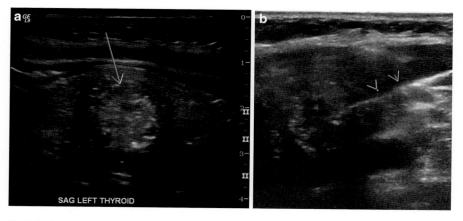

Fig. 1 Left thyroid nodule. A preliminary sonogram (**a**) demonstrates a ~2 cm left thyroid nodule (*large arrow*) containing numerous echogenic foci consistent with microcalcifications. Ultrasound-guided biopsy (**b**) demonstrates the needle (*small arrows*) entering the nodule. The cytologic diagnosis was papillary carcinoma

General Complications and Management

- Transient post-procedural hoarseness may occur and usually resolves within 2 h, presumably due to lidocaine effects on the laryngeal nerves. Permanent hoarseness after thyroid biopsy is very rare and can be managed by referral to a head and neck surgeon.
- Patients may be advised to present to the nearest emergency room if shortness of breath or difficulty swallowing develop. This is exceedingly uncommon.

Tools for Biopsy

Needle Types

- Fine-needle aspiration: 25 gauge 5 cm long needles
- Core biopsy: 20 gauge 6 cm long core biopsy needle

Specimen Handling

- FNA specimens are placed in a cytological fixing agent – either ethyl alcohol for slides or 25% methyl alcohol for in-solution fixation.
- Core biopsies may be placed in saline or formalin depending on local pathology laboratory preference.
- If a parathyroid neoplasm is thought likely, it is helpful to send one of the specimens for a parathyroid hormone assay.

FNA Versus Core

- FNA and core have been shown to have equivalent diagnostic accuracy for the characterization of thyroid nodules. Because of a theoretically greater risk of complication with core biopsy, most practitioners perform FNA first. If the FNA is not diagnostic, then FNA and core biopsy can be performed at the second visit. This will yield a diagnosis in ~85% of cases.

Alternatives

- Palpable nodules may be biopsied without imaging guidance using direct palpation for guidance.
- Imaging guidance is essential for the biopsy of impalpable nodules.

Key Points

> Thyroid biopsy is a relatively safe procedure that may be performed on an outpatient basis without conscious sedation.
> Indications for thyroid nodule biopsy vary across practitioners and have not yet been definitively established.
> Characteristics that may lead to biopsy include size >10–15 mm, microcalcifications, AP nodule diameter greater than transverse diameter, interval growth, intranodular vascularity, FDG avidity, and sestamibi avidity.

Suggested Reading

1. Cappelli C, Castellano M, Pirola I, et al. Thyroid nodule shape suggests malignancy. *Eur J Endocrinol/Eur Federation Endocrine Soc.* 2006;155(1):27-31.
2. Kim EK, Park CS, Chung WY, et al. New sonographic criteria for recommending fine-needle aspiration biopsy of nonpalpable solid nodules of the thyroid. *AJR Am J Roentgenol.* 2002;178(3):687-691.
3. Morris LF, Ragavendra N, Yeh MW. Evidence-based assessment of the role of ultrasonography in the management of benign thyroid nodules. *World J Surg.* 2008;32(7):1253-1263.
4. Pothier DD, Narula AA. Should we apply suction during fine needle cytology of thyroid lesions? A systematic review and meta-analysis. *Ann R Coll Surg Engl.* 2006;88(7):643-645.

Prostate Biopsy

Melina Pectasides

Clinical Features

- Prostate cancer is the most common noncutaneous cancer in men, and the second leading cause of male cancer mortality.
- No routine screening guidelines for prostate cancer have been established. Digital rectal examination (DRE) and serum prostate-specific antigen (PSA) levels should be offered to asymptomatic men 40 years of age or older who wish to be screened with an estimated life expectancy of more than 10 years. Determination of future screening intervals is based upon the first DRE findings and PSA levels.
- Ninety-five percent of prostate cancers are adenocarcinomas that develop in the acini of the prostatic ducts.
- Cancer is found in the peripheral zone of the prostate in approximately 60-70%, in the transition zone in 10-20%, and in the central zone in 5-10%.

Diagnostic Evaluation

Clinical

- The digital rectal exam has a high false-negative rate of 25–45% and only 20% of palpable lesions are curable.

Laboratory

- PSA, in conjunction with DRE, is used for early diagnosis of prostate cancer and for monitoring for disease recurrence. Men with a PSA level greater than 2.5 ng/mL have a 20% chance of finding prostate cancer at biopsy, and this increases to 50% if the PSA is greater than 10 ng/mL.

M. Pectasides
Radiology Department, Massachusetts General Hospital, Boston, MA, USA

D.A. Gervais and T. Sabharwal (eds.),
Interventional Radiology Procedures in Biopsy and Drainage,
DOI: 10.1007/978-1-84800-899-1_12, © Springer-Verlag London Limited 2011

Imaging

- The established radiological sign of prostate cancer is the hypoechoic nodule on transrectal ultrasound (TRUS). However, the positive predictive value of the hypoechoic lesion in the average urologic population is low, ranging between 18% and 53%. Moreover, up to 30% of all prostate cancers are isoechoic.
- Since detection and localization of prostate tumors using greyscale ultrasound is poor, TRUS is mainly used to guide systematic biopsies.

Indications

- The decision to proceed to prostate biopsy is based primarily on PSA and DRE results. However, one should take into account multiple factors, including free and total PSA, patient age, PSA velocity, PSA density, family history, ethnicity, prior biopsy history and comorbidities.

Contraindications

- Contraindications to prostate biopsy include acute painful perianal disorders, bleeding diathesis, acute prostatitis, and severe immunosuppression.
- Transrectal ultrasound-guided prostate biopsy is impossible in patients lacking a rectum, as those who have undergone ano-rectal resection. In those cases, transgluteal biopsy under CT guidance is performed.

Patient Preparation

- The patient should discontinue oral anticoagulants approximately 7–10 days prior to the procedure.
- Coagulation parameters are not routinely checked unless there is a reason for them to be abnormal. For patients on warfarin or with an underlying coagulopathy, International Normalized Ratio (INR) should be corrected to below 1.5 and platelets above 50,000.
- Patients receive oral antibiotics on the day prior, the day of, and for 5 days after the procedure. Agents commonly used are oral fluoroquinolones, e.g., levofloxacin.

Anatomy

- The prostate is split into four distinct zones: the central zone, peripheral zone, and transition zone, as well as the fibromuscular stroma.
- In young men, the peripheral zone comprises 75% of the volume of the prostate. After the age of 40, benign prostatic hyperplasia begins in the transition zone.
- Prostate cancer is located in the peripheral zone in approximately 70% of patients.

Equipment

- Transrectal ultrasound transducer with needle guide
- 18 gauge cutting needle biopsy gun

Pre-procedure Medications

- A cleansing enema on the morning of the procedure is optional.
- One dose of parenteral antibiotics is given just prior to the procedure. This usually is a dose of gentamycin 80 mg. It is given IM; if the patient has prosthetic cardiac valves or joints, it has to be given IV.
- The necessity for periprocedural pain control is debatable. There are many methods used; the most popular approach being the peri-prostatic nerve block. The nerves can be blocked with lidocaine injection at the hyperechoic fat pad that demarcates the junction of the seminal vesicles and the prostate bilaterally.

Procedure

- The patient is placed in the left lateral decubitus position with hips and knees flexed.
- The transducer is inserted and the prostate volume is measured. The exam is started at the base of the prostate and extends to the apex, with imaging in both tranverse and sagittal planes.
- Lidocaine anesthesia is performed with a long spinal needle (22 gauge) and TRUS guidance at the seminal vesicle – prostate junction bilaterally.
- Currently, the originally sextant biopsy scheme is replaced by extended schemes, using more cores directed at the peripheral zone. The biopsy gun is guided to take five peripheral zone biopsies and one central biopsy on either side, starting at the base and ending at the apex (Figs. 1 and 2).
- Any hypoechoic suspicious nodules should also be separately biopsied.
- Applying constant gentle forward pressure with the transducer during the biopsy flattens the rectal wall, reducing discomfort and bleeding.
- The specimen is placed in 10% formalin with correct labeling of side and region of biopsy.

Immediate Post-Procedure Care

- A rectal examination may be performed after the biopsy with pressure applied to the prostate.
- The patient is advised to remain lying for 15 min post procedure and may be discharged if stable.

In patients lacking a rectum, a CT-guided transgluteal prostate biopsy may be performed (Fig. 3).

Fig. 1 Transrectal ultrasound-guided prostate biopsy of the right and left prostatic peripheral zone

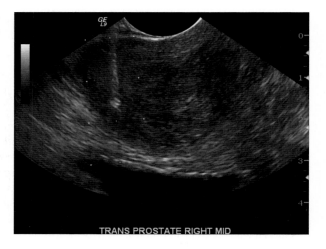

Fig. 2 Transrectal ultrasound-guided prostate biopsy of the right and left prostatic peripheral zone

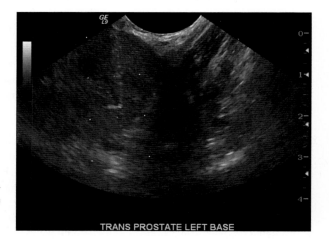

- The patient needs to fast for 6 h before the procedure.
- Antibiotic prophylaxis is not routinely used.
- Intravenous conscious sedation is used with midazolam and fentanyl. Oxygen saturation, blood pressure, and heart rate and rhythm are monitored throughout the procedure.
- The patient is placed prone on the CT table.
- Lidocaine infiltration of the skin and soft tissues is performed. Peri-prostatic lidocaine is not necessary in this scenario.

Fig. 3 CT-guided transgluteal prostate biopsy in a patient lacking a rectum post lower anterior resection. Bilateral guiding needles are poised to allow passage of biopsy needles into peripheral gland

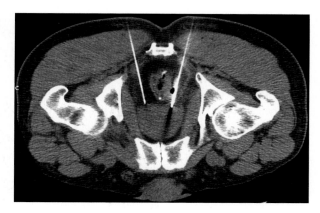

- Under CT guidance and using a transgluteal approach, two 17-gauge coaxial systems are advanced to the near surface of the peripheral zone of the prostate on each side. The 17-gauge needle is manipulated to guide the core caudally, cranially, medially and laterally in the prostate and biopsies are taken at the apex, midway between the apex and base and at the base. Twelve 18-gauge cores are obtained.
- A post-procedure CT is performed to rule out any immediate complication.

Immediate Post-Procure Care CT-guided Transgluteal Prostate Biopsy

- The patient may be discharged 3 h after the procedure, if stable.

Complications

- Infections: Febrile urinary tract infection, bacteremia or acute prostatitis. Rare cases of fatal septicemia have been reported. Treatment is achieved with oral or intravenous antibiotics depending on the severity of the infection.
- Bleeding: Rectal bleeding, hematuria or hematospermia. Usually bleeding is self-limiting and should resolve within 1 week. More significant rectal bleeding may require anoscopic intervention.
- Acute urinary retention has been described, especially in patients with significant BPH.

Alternative Procedures/Future Directions

- Contrast-enhanced transrectal ultrasound: Infusion of intravenous microbubble ultrasound contrast agents can amplify flow signals within the microvasculature of prostate tumors, thus making them more conspicuous and allowing for more accurate biopsy sampling of the prostate.

Key Points

> Antibiotic prophylaxis is needed for transrectal US-guided prostate biopsy.
> Extended biopsy schemes should be performed with five peripheral and one central core on either side of the prostate, with additional cores for any hypoechoic lesions detected.
> Transgluteal CT-guided prostate biopsy can be performed in patients lacking a rectum.
> Most common complications include infections and bleeding (rectal, hematuria, hematospermia).

Suggested Reading

1. Campbell-Walsh urology, 9th ed. /editor-in-chief, Alan J. Wein; editors, Louis R. Kavoussi et al.
2. Raja J et al. Current status of transrectal ultrasound-guided prostate biopsy in the diagnosis of prostate cancer. *Clin Radiol.* 2006;61(2):142-153.
3. Eichler K et al. Diagnostic value of systematic biopsy methods in the investigation of prostate cancer: a systematic review. *J Urol.* 2006;175(5):1605-1612.
4. Pallwein L et al. Ultrasound of prostate cancer: recent advances. *Eur Radiol.* 2008;18(4):707-715. Epub 2007 Oct 16.
5. AUA (2009) Prostate-specific antigen best practice statement: 2009 update. American Urological Society.
6. Wink M et al. Contrast-enhanced ultrasound and prostate cancer; a multicentre European research coordination project. *Eur Urol.* 2008;54(5):982-992. Epub 2008 Jun 20.
7. Cantwell CP et al. Prostate biopsy after ano-rectal resection: value of CT-guided trans-gluteal biopsy. *Eur Radiol.* 2008;18(4):738-742. Epub 2008 Jan 10.

Drainage of Abdominal Fluid Collections

Shuvro Roy-Choudhury

Percutaneous abscess drainage (PAD) is now standard therapy for patients with intraabdominal abscess who do not have other indications for surgery. The vast majority of collections or abscesses can be managed with an appropriately sized and positioned catheter. This section will deal with some general principles of abscess drainage as well as look into some specific locations like perihepatic (subphrenic and subhepatic), gall bladder bed, splenic bed, lesser sac, paracolic, and retroperitoneal abscesses.

Clinical Features: Most abscesses are (a) postoperative, (b) consequence of acute inflammatory abdominal condition like cholecystitis, appendicitis, diverticulitis with or without perforation, (c) due to associated inflammatory bowel disease, (d) due to trauma, or (e) due to tuberculosis.

- Right subphrenic collections are usually related to gastro-hepato-biliary surgery and bile leaks.
- Left subphrenic collections are usually related to gastric, splenic, colonic, or pancreatic surgery and pathology.
- Paracolic collections are related to bowel (often diverticular or Crohn's) or appendiceal pathologies.
- Retroperitoneal collections are related to renal, ureteric, duodenal, pancreatic, bowel, paraaortic, or paraspinal pathologies.

Diagnostic Evaluation

- *Clinical*: This is the most important criteria for referral for PAD. Patients feel unwell, have swinging pyrexia, and have associated abdominal pain and tenderness.
- *Laboratory*: CRP and leucocytosis reflects the degree of sepsis and is useful for decision making.
- *Imaging*: Clinical suspicion of an intraabdominal collection/abscess is often confirmed with imaging usually with CT or US.

S. Roy-Choudhury
Radiology Department, Heart of England NHS Foundation Trust, Birmingham, UK

D.A. Gervais and T. Sabharwal (eds.),
Interventional Radiology Procedures in Biopsy and Drainage,
DOI: 10.1007/978-1-84800-899-1_13, © Springer-Verlag London Limited 2011

- Planning:
  - Assess pre-intervention imaging (preferably CT) in multiplanar formats to identify anatomical location of abscess and plan guiding modality and access route.
  - Assess abscess content for guidance on size of catheter required. It is desirable to distinguish between phlegmonous change (likely unsuccessful drainage) and an abscess with an enhancing wall, although sometimes a needle aspirate is necessary to differentiate between the two.
- Choosing the modality for guidance:
  - US: easier, cheaper, provides real-time guidance, ideal for superficial collections or for angled access, and provides more information about abscess content.
  - CT with or without CT fluoroscopy: Safer, avoids bowel, and better for deeper abscesses and those which contain gas. Gas locules deep within collection that has not risen to the top implies thick material or loculation.
  - Fluoroscopy – useful, underutilized – particularly for repositioning drains (using wires and torquing catheters) to drain difficult locules or to finalize drain position after US or CT-guided access. Also useful to perform abscessograms

Indications/contraindications: These are relative and depends on the acuteness and severity of the sepsis.

- Generally, an abscess <4 cm should not be considered for PAD (as these may well heal on conservative management) unless the patient is septic attributable to the collection.
- Multiple or multiloculated abscesses may be better dealt with by surgery.

Patient Preparation

- Oral gastrograffin to opacify bowel for interloop abscesses, particularly in thin patients if procedure is CT-guided.

Broad spectrum antibiotics should be administered intravenously if the patient is not already receiving antibiotic therapy.

Relevant Anatomy

Normal anatomy: It is vital to learn the peritoneal reflections and the potential spaces for abdominal abscesses to collect. The perihepatic space is a dependent part of the supine abdomen and hence abscesses often occur here. The negative hydrostatic pressure, particularly during inspiration allows transcoelomic migration of fluid to this region, more to the right side, due to the shallow left paracolic gutter and the obstruction by the left phrenico-colic ligament.

The liver is invested by the visceral peritoneum except at the bare area, the gall bladder bed, and the porta hepatis whence it gets reflected to the diaphragm, ligamentum teres, and the lesser omentum, respectively. The resulting perihepatic spaces are divided by the peritoneal ligaments like the falciform, coronary, and triangular ligaments (Fig. 1). The spaces are (a) right subphrenic, (b) left subphrenic, (c) left subhepatic, and (d) right subhepatic, or hepatorenal pouch of Morrisson which communicates with the lesser sac through the Foramen of Winslow. The right-sided spaces freely communicate. The subhepatic spaces communicate via the paracolic spaces to the pelvic peritoneum.

Aberrant anatomy: Be careful about collateral vessels in portal hypertension

Equipment: Practices vary and it is vital to get acquainted with the kit used in your unit. Most drainages are preceeded by aspiration when using the commonly used Seldinger technique. Drainage can be performed without aspiration using the "one step" trocar technique (see below).

For aspiration: Sterile pack, local anesthesia set,18–22G needle (Angiocath, Kellet, Chiba, etc.), 20 mL syringe, scalpel, sterile US probe cover, specimen pots.

For drainage: In addition to above – a selection of guidewires, dilators, and drains with appropriate connectors, drainage bags, and skin securing devices. Locking pigtail drains are preferred. 6–8 F drains are used for clear fluid, 8–10 F for thin pus, 10–12 F for thick pus and 12–22 F for abscesses with debris. Occasionally a biliary manipulation catheter, hydrophillic guidewire, or Neff set will be used.

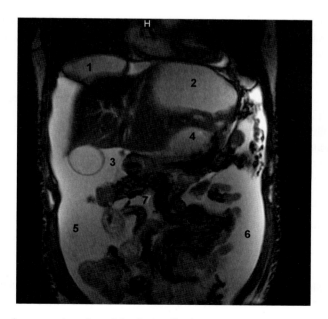

Fig. 1 Peritoneal spaces where intraabdominal collections occur.The right (1) and left (2) subphrenic spaces are separated by the falciform ligament. The right (3) and left (4) subhepatic spaces communicate with the respective subphrenic spaces superiorly and the right (5) and left (6) paracolic spaces inferiorly. Interloop abscesses collect between intraperitoneal bowel loops (7). Note the subtle difference in signal intensity in this patient with acute pancreatitis between free fluid (1 and 3) and a left subphrenic and subhepatic abscess (2 and 4)

Pre-procedure medications: Patient are usually on antibiotics. Sedoanalgesia as per local practice.

Procedure

Planning an Access Route

- Generally choose the safest, straightest, shortest route to the largest part of the abscess (cf subphrenic abscess, see below). Think about patient comfort.
- Plan to place the catheter in the most dependent part of the abscess.
- Plan such that there is potential to withdraw the catheter to drain more superficial parts of the abscess.
- Aim for long axis of collection if possible and change angle of approach as necessary.
- If significantly angled access – use US or angle the CT gantry.
- Some loops of bowel can be displaced by compression with US probe during access.
- Use color doppler to avoid vessels. Hydrodissection can also be used to create a safe access.
- Accessing subphrenic collections can be difficult due to the risk of pleural transgression and resulting pleural infection. It is best to choose a low (subcostal if possible) anterior extrapleural access. A combination of US and fluoroscopy can be very useful in this setting. However, transpleural access is sometimes inevitable and in fact has been shown to be equally effective.
- Surgical drain tracts can be used for access.
- It is usually safe to transgress liver or stomach for life threatening subhepatic, paraduodenal, gall bladder bed, or lesser sac abscesses. Avoid large liver vessels, dilated bile ducts, gallbladder, or large perigastric vessels.
- For the completely inaccessible interloop abscess – consider aspirating abscess to dryness transgressing bowel with a 20G needle to provide a sample.

Performing the Procedure

Technique

One step technique (Trocar technique): Only for superficial collections and small-sized drains. After aseptic preparation and local anesthetic infiltration (as close to the abscess wall as possible), a catheter mounted on a stiffener/stylet and a central sharp needle is inserted directly under imaging guidance to penetrate the anterior wall of the abscess. The central sharp needle is removed and a small amount of fluid is aspirated to confirm entry. The outer catheter is then moved further in the abscess while the central stylet is held in place.

Two step/Seldinger technique: Standard practice and usually follows a diagnostic aspiration performed under US or CT guidance. Choose drain size after aspiration. Depending on access needle size, use a 0.035 guidewire or use 0.018 wire and Neff set and upsize to 0.035 system. This track is then dilated to the desired size of the intended drain. The central sharp needle is discarded and the catheter mounted on the stylet is inserted coaxially over the wire into the abscess. In complex or angulated access fluoroscopy may be useful along with wires and catheters to obtain better position with a drain.

At this stage position may be confirmed by US, CT, or a limited abcessogram. A three way connector is attached and as much as possible of the offending material is aspirated. Bloody aspirate indicates apposition of walls. The drain is connected to a bag and secured by sutures or adhesive dressings (several commercial ones available) or both!

Ensure that the specimens are sent to the laboratory.

Tips

- If drainage is contemplated, do not aspirate too much fluid.
- Use a curved wire – occasionally even the blunt end of a straight wire will penetrate the posterior wall of a thin abscess.
- Angle access if possible so as to avoid hitting the posterior wall of the abscess at right angles, particularly for shallow ones.
- Use a dilator only to penetrate the anterior wall (mentally measure this!) – too deep dilatation can kink the wire or perforate the abscess.
- In larger catheters one can increase the number of sideholes to drain a longer segment.
- Biloculated collections can be drained by inserting an internal-external drain (Fig. 2) or withdrawing catheter after deeper locule has been drained.
- Consider putting two (or three) drains in large or loculated abscesses.
- Consider a peel away sheath when inserting large catheters and there is a risk of kinking.
- Mechanical disruption of thin loculi is possible with a pigtail catheter.
- Be wary of resolving hematoma or necrotic tumor simulating an abscess – if in doubt, aspirate first. If material is not aspiratable, consider a core biopsy.
- Image the collection immediately after drainage to make sure there are no undrained locules.

Endpoint: A comfortable patient leaving the interventional suite with an almost completely drained abscess and the drain catheter still connected!

Immediate post-procedure care: Send a nursing post-care form with standard instructions to monitor pulse, blood pressure, temperature and prescribed analgesia. Position the patient to make the drain dependent. IV fluids may be required.

Follow-Up and Post-Procedure

Medications: These include analgesia and antibiotics.

Post-procedure patient and drain care: This should ideally be supervised by the interventional team.

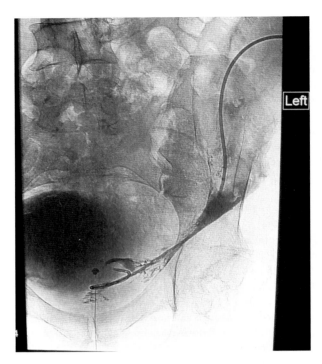

Fig. 2 Use of fluoroscopy: Axial CT image had shown a left paracolic abscess communicating with a further interloop abscess through a narrow channel in a patient with inflammatory bowel disease (not shown). The superficial locule has been accessed under ultrasound guidance. Under fluoroscopy a wire has been manipulated into the deeper locule. An internal-external drain with side holes to drain both locules has been placed. An alternative strategy could be to drain the deeper locule followed by withdrawal of the drain to the more superficial locule

- The patients temperature, laboratory data (gram stain, cultures, WCC) is monitored daily along with the drainage amount (q shift).
- The exit site, catheter condition, and integrity of retention are monitored.
- Catheter irrigation is supervised.
- Communication with, and educating ward nurses and clinical team is critical.

Further intervention is necessary when:

- Fever persists – repeat imaging or perform drainogram under fluoroscopy. Repositioning or further catheters may be necessary.
- Catheter has fallen out: If the tract is a few days old it is usually possible to reenter the tract with a catheter and a hydrophillic guide wire.
- Catheter is blocked or kinked: Most kinks are outside the body – in the dressings! Flushing with saline or manipulating with a guide wire usually clears a blocked cath-

teter. If reinserting the wire is difficult, one can put an oversheath over the catheter after removing the hub and replace a new catheter.

Tips to drain viscous collection

- Gently flush drain with 20 mL saline two to three times a day
- Use a sump drain
- Use urokinase or tPA – the former at 50,000 IU in saline thrice daily with 15 min clamp and release (Haaga protocol). Urokinase is not approved by the FDA – use tPA instead: 4–6 mg tPA in 25 mL of normal saline instilled thrice daily, catheter clamped for 30 min, then drained, for 2–3 days. This cycle can be repeated.

Abscess–Fistula Complex

- Low-output and high-output fistulas can prolong abscess drainage.
- Low output (<100 mL/day) generally occur with large bowel and usually heal with drainage of the associated abscess.
- High-output fistulas should be suspected if persistemt high outputs >200 mL/day occur or if output increases after 3–4 days of drainage.
- High-output fistulas are with small bowel and can be more difficult to treat.
- Principles include: draining the abscess, diverting the proximal bowel, bowel rest, managing sepsis, relplacing fluid and electrolytes, and IV feeding.
- Other factors that influence fistula healing include; distal obstruction, bowel integrity at fistula site, and immune status of the patient.
- Bowel diversion can be achieved by NG suction or by manipulating a separate catheter through the abscess into the bowel. This catheter can be left until a mature track forms around it and is then withdrawn slowly.
- Note if there is a biliary/duodenal fistula, the biliary tree should be drained also.
- Quoted success rates for abscess/fistula drainage vary from 66% to 82%.
- In general, if the fistula has not healed by 6 weeks, surgery may be necessary.

Removal of Drain

- Resolution of fever/leucocytosis
- Daily drainage <20 mL/day and source of sepsis controlled.
- Imaging shows resolution of abscess.
- Catheter-related problems like malposition, kinking, or blockage.
- If transpleural access is used in subphrenic abscess, ensure that the tract is mature before removal to prevent contamination of pleural cavity. A tractogram can be performed before removal.

Results: PAD is usually regarded to be safe and effective alternative to surgery with a higher success rate, lower complication rate and morbidity, and a shorter hospital stay. Success rates of 62.4% to 96% have been reported – most of these series are from 1980s and 1990s. Lang et al. reported 90/119 drainage procedures with a curative intent and 15/17 with a temporizing intent was successful. A mortality rate of 1.4% and complication rate of 5% was reported. With state of the art drain care and tPA instillation, even complex, recalcitrant abscesses can be cured in upto 89% cases.

Causes of Failure

- Persisting fistulous communication – perform drainogram to confirm
- Early removal of drain – after acute sepsis subsides. It is preferable to image prior to removal if in doubt
- Collection is loculated – consider multiple drains, tPA, or surgery
- Fungal infection
- Crohn's disease – PAD first line, but, one-third require surgery
- Misplaced catheter
- Inappropriate site of entry

Alternative Therapies: The principle alternative therapy is surgery (if associated with large visceral perforation, failed PAD, multiloculation, or multiple abscesses) or conservative treatment with antibiotics (if smaller than 4 cm, low-grade pyrexia and/or patient clinically recovering).

Complications:	Peritonitis	2%
	Septicaemia and bacteraemia	1–5%
	Haematoma and vascular injury	2%
	Pneumothorax	
	Pleural effusion	2–10%
	Empyema	
	Bowel injury	1%

How to Avoid

- Avoid perforating the posterior wall of the abscess
- Do not flush too vigorously – this may allow venous contamination and septicaemia
- Avoid transgressing the pleura. Allow tract to mature before drain removal
- Use color doppler to avoid vessels

Key Points

> Almost all intraabdominal abscesses are accessible percutaneously.
> Transgressing solid organs and occasionally hollow organs is acceptable to gain access and can be done with surprising little morbidity
> Critical assessment of pre-procedure imaging to plan access
> Familiarize with the drainage kit, securing device, etc.
> Fluoroscopy can be invaluable. Combination of modalities can often be useful.
> Post-procedure catheter care is as important as inserting the catheter.
> Subphrenic abscesses can be difficult because of potential trangression of pleura. Use a combination of ultrasound and fluoroscopy and a low anterior access.

Suggested Reading

1. Maher MM, Gervais DA, Kalra MK, et al. The inaccessible or undrainable abscess: how to drain it. *Radiographics*. 2004;24(3):717-735. Review.
2. Lambiase RE, Deyoe L, Cronan JJ, Dorfman GS. Percutaneous drainage of 335 consecutive abscesses: results of primary drainage with 1-year follow-up. *Radiology*. 1992;184(1): 167-179.
3. Bakal CW, Sacks D, Burke DR, et al. Society of Interventional Radiology Standards of Practice Committee. Quality improvement guidelines for adult percutaneous abscess and fluid drainage. *J Vasc Interv Radiol*. 2003;14(9 Pt 2):S223-S225.
4. Gervais DA, Ho CH, O'Neill MJ, Arellano RS, Hahn PF, Mueller PR. Recurrent abdominal and pelvic abscesses: incidence, results of repeated percutaneous drainage, and underlying causes in 956 drainages. *AJR Am J Roentgenol*. 2004;182(2):463-466.

Drainage of Pelvic Fluid Collections

Ajay K. Singh

Clinical Features

Image-guided catheter drainage has become the treatment of choice for most pelvic abscesses developing secondary to recent surgery, pelvic inflammatory disease, perforated appendicitis, inflammatory bowel disease, and perforated diverticulitis. Percutaneous abscess drainage is curative in more than 80% of the cases.[1] In other cases, percutaneous abscess drainage may play a role in managing critically ill patients improving their sepsis while they get better in order to undergo definitive surgery.

Diagnostic Evaluation

Clinical

- Fever.
- May have sepsis with tachycardia and hypotension.
- Large collections may cause symptoms from mass effect such as pain, obstruction, and bloating.

Laboratory

- CBC may show leukocytosis and left shift.
- Elderly debilitated patients may fail to express fever or leukocytosis.
- Check INR and platelets and correct coagulopathy if needed.

A.K. Singh
Department of Radiology, Massachusetts General Hospital, Boston, MA, USA

D.A. Gervais and T. Sabharwal (eds.),
Interventional Radiology Procedures in Biopsy and Drainage,
DOI: 10.1007/978-1-84800-899-1_14, © Springer-Verlag London Limited 2011

Imaging

- Pelvic fluid collection on CT with well-defined enhancing rim characteristic of abscess.
- May have inflammatory changes adjacent to collection.
- May have inflammatory changes of diseased adjacent bowel in cases of appendicitis, diverticulitis, inflammatory bowel disease.
- Review imaging to confirm diagnosis of abscess and to plan drainage.
- Review imaging to identify normal and abnormal adjacent bowel loops.

Indications

- To drain infected fluid as a necessary adjunct to antibiotics
- To relieve sepsis
- To relieve symptoms due to mass effect of collection

Contraindications

- Lack of safe access route
- Irreversible coagulopathy

Alternative Therapies

- Surgical drainage is performed in patients with other indications for surgery (e.g., peritonitis, small bowel obstruction) or in those with no access route.
- Surgical drainage may be necessary in cases of failed percutaneous drainage.
- Treatment with antibiotics alone can be considered for small abscess.

Patient Preparation

- IV access and 8 hour fasting for safe sedation.
- Antibiotics for patients with infection; if already on antibiotics, routine dosing may be adequate.
- Pre-procedural antibiotics for patients drained via a transrectal or transvaginal approach regardless of whether the collection is infected or not.
- Patients presenting for drainage of noninfected collections where the drainage path does not transgress bowel do not need antibiotics.

Relevant Anatomy

Normal

Loops of bowel may be nearby anywhere in the pelvis. Laterally, bone and ileac vessels may impede an access route. Bladder and bowel may limit percutaneous access to deep pelvic abscesses. Uterus and adnexa may also limit access. Anatomy is reviewed on diagnostic imaging prior to drainage.

Aberrant/Altered

Post surgical anatomy can be misleading unless correlated with surgical history.
- Femoral to femoral artery bypass grafts low in the pelvis or axillofemoral grafts coursing laterally should be avoided.
- Augmented bladders or reservoirs for urological devices may look like fluid collections and be incorrectly interpreted as abscesses.
- Blind ends of end-to-side bowel anastomoses may simulate small fluid collections.
- Diversion of enteral flow to a proximal ostomy may often result in many normal or abnormal loops of pelvic bowel remaining unopacified on CT.
- Anastomoses can be identified by searching for the radio-opaque suture line. Abscesses from leaking anastomoses are typically nearby.

Equipment

- 8–14 French Pigtail Drainage Catheter.
- 16–20 French nonpigtail drainage catheters for extremely viscous material in larger spaces.
- For trocar technique, 20 G guiding needle of appropriate length.
- For Seldinger technique, 0.035″ or 0.038″ stiff wire and dilators. May need to over dilate 1 or 2 French sizes compared to catheter.
- Standard drainage bags, connector tubing form catheter to bag, three-way stopcock.

Procedure

Technique

- *Tandem Trocar Technique*: 18–21 gauge needle placed into abscess and confirmed to be in abscess with imaging. Trocar catheter is then advanced via an adjacent skin nick 5–15 mm away from the needle skin entry perfectly parallel to the needle in order to enter the abscess. Once in the abscess, the catheter is advanced off the trocar.

- *Seldinger Technique*: 18–21 guage needle placed into abscess and inner stylet removed to allow guidewire placement into abscess. Tract is then serially dilated and the catheter is deployed over the wire. Tract may need dilatation 1 or 2 French above catheter size.
- Neither technique has been proved superior or safer than the other. Technique choices are usually a matter of operator preference.

Planning an Access Route

- Review of diagnostic imaging, most commonly CT but sometimes MR, is critical to access route planning.
- Collections superficial to the abdominal muscles can often be drained with ultrasound guidance using an anterior or anterolateral approach.
- Collections deep to the superficial abdominal muscles can often be drained via an anterior approach. This may require CT guidance to identify the abscess as separate from bowel.
- Deep pelvic abscesses may be difficult or impossible to drain anteriorly.
- Deep pelvic abscesses can often be drained using a transgluteal approach through the greater sciatic foramen.
- Proximity of a collection to the vaginal fornices or to the low rectum may render a transvaginal or transrectal approach feasible.
- Low collections can sometimes be drained via a transperineal approach.

Routes of Pelvic Drainage (Fig. 1a)

Transgluteal Approach

- Anatomy of greater sciatic foramen:
  — Margins: sacrospinous ligament inferiorly, ischium anteriorly, and ilium superiorly.
  — The piriformis muscle passes through the center of the greater sciatic foramen, and is posterior to the sacral plexus, which gives rise to sciatic nerve inferiorly.
  — The superior and inferior gluteal arteries and veins cross the foramen in the most cephalic aspect.
  — The major vessels and neural structures are located cephalad to sacrospinous ligament.[4]
- Technique (Figs. 1 and 2):
  — Positioning: Prone, prone oblique, or decubitus.
  — Mostly performed under CT guidance.
  — Ideal approach: Place the catheter as close to the sacrum as possible (to avoid sciatic nerve injury), at the level of the sacrospinous ligament.

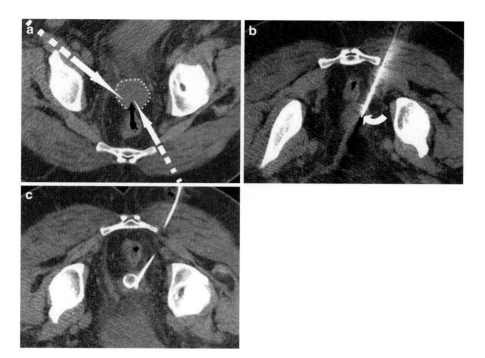

Fig. 1 Routes of drainage of a pelvic collection. (**a**) Axial noncontrast CT of the pelvis demonstrating a loculated collection in the rectovesical pouch. The anterior approach (*right arrow*) for drainage passes through the right iliopsoas muscle while the posterior approach (*left arrow*) through the left greater sciatic foramen passes just lateral to the sacrum. Another approach of treatment in this male patient would be a transrectal approach (*black arrow*). (**b**) Axial contrast CT obtained during the percutaneous drainage using Trocar technique, shows the drainage catheter tip (*curved arrow*) in the pelvic collection. (**c**) Axial contrast CT after deployment of the 10 F pigtail catheter shows complete resolution of the pelvic collection

- — Infra-piriformis approach preferred when possible to avoid injury to gluteal vessels and sacral plexus located anterior to the piriformis muscle.
- — Trocar or Seldinger technique used to place a pigtail drainage catheter. If collection is sterile than an 18–20 gauge needle may be used for aspiration, without drainage.
- Up to 20% of patients have catheter-related pain lasting more than 24 h.

Anterior Approach

- CT guidance: To better assess the bowel loops and deeper abscesses.
- Catheter size, most often 8–14 French.
- Often made difficult by intervening bowel, vascular, or osseous structures.

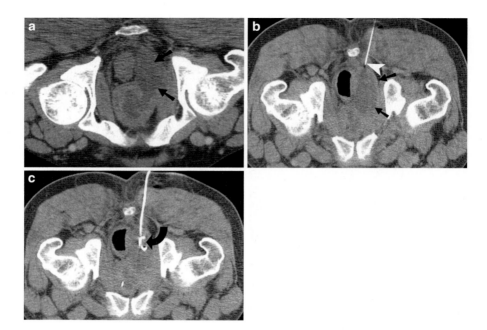

Fig. 2 Pelvic abscess drainage with Trocar technique. (**a**) Axial contrast-enhanced CT shows prostatic abscess with rupture component (*arrows*) next to obturator internus muscle. (**b**) Noncontrast CT during procedure shows a 20 G needle (*arrowhead*) placed in the direction of the abscess (*arrow*). (**c**) Noncontrast CT shows a pigtail drainage catheter (*curved arrow*) deployed parallel to the guiding needle

- Angled gantry approach may be required to avoid bowel loops.
- Trocar or Seldinger (Fig. 3) technique used.

Transrectal or Transvaginal Access (Figs. 4 and 5)

- Performed under US guidance.[5]
- Transrectal route is better tolerated than transvaginal route.
- Transvaginal route not used in pediatric patients.

Transperineal Approach

- Used for deep pelvic collection, e.g., collections after abdominoperineal resection.
- May be successfully performed in patients who cannot undergo conventional transabdominal, transvaginal, or transrectal catheter drainage.[6]
- Can be performed with ultrasound or CT guidance.
- Tissues are typically tough to penetrate.

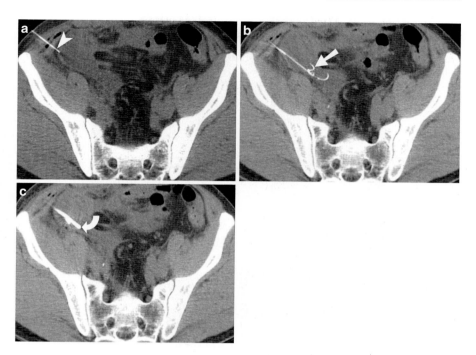

Fig. 3 Seldinger's technique. (**a**) Axial noncontrast CT shows a right lower collection with a micropuncture needle tip (*arrowhead*) at its periphery. (**b**) Axial noncontrast CT shows a 0.018 wire (*arrow*) passed through the needle, in to the collection. A sheath is placed over the 0.018 wire and then the micropuncture wire is exchanged for an Amplatz wire. (**c**) Axial noncontrast CT shows a pigtail drainage catheter placed in the collection, over an Amplatz wire

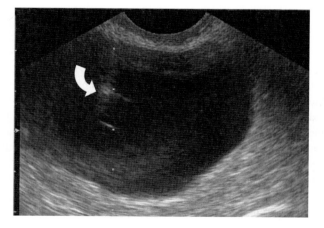

Fig. 4 Transvaginal needle aspiration. Transvaginal US shows a 20 G aspiration needle (*curved arrow*) within the pelvic fluid collection

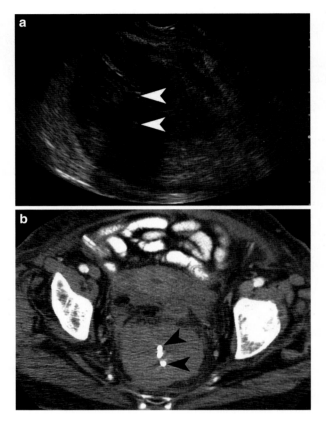

Fig. 5 Transrectal catheter drainage. (**a**) Transrectal US shows pigtail drainage catheter (*arrowheads*) within the pelvic abscess. (**b**) Noncontrast axial CT shows a drainage catheter (*arrowheads*) within the pelvic abscess

Endpoint

- Imaging after placement of abcess catheter and removal of contents ideally shows collapsed collection.
- Complete drainage can sometimes be enhanced by irrigation with small quantities of 0.9% saline solution making sure to keep the injected volume lower than the volume initially removed from the cavity in order to minimize bacteremia and sepsis.
- Large collections may require more than one catheter for complete drainage.
- If a portion of the collection persists with cathether in good position, it may drain with time.
- However, if most of the collection persists, consider adjunctive thrombolytics such as tPA.

Results

Percutaneous abscess drainage is successful in 80–90% of cases.
The determinants of high success rate with catheter drainage are:

- Postoperative
- Not pancreatic
- Not infected with yeast[1]

The determinants of poor success with catheter drainage are:

- Bowel communication or other fistula
- Multiple abscesses
- Crohn's disease
- Pancreatic abscess
- Infected tumor
- Infected clot
- *Complications*: Complications are rare (<5% in most series) and include hemorrhage, bacteremia, transient worsening of sepsis, organ injury, bowel injury, and superinfection.

Follow Up

Catheter Management

The catheter is left to gravity drainage and flushed with 0.9% saline solution every 8–12 h to maintain catheter patency.

Antibiotics are continued and adjusted as necessary based on the culture and sensitivity results of the abscess contents.

The criteria for catheter removal are:

- Most important is the clinical status of the patient. Successful drainage is usually associated with an increased sense of well being.
- Defervescence.
- Improvement in leukocytosis.
- Drainage <10–20 mL/day
- Absence of catheter malposition, blockage, or kinking; When present these may necessitate replacing or repositioning the catheter if residual abscess remains.
- Imaging features: Demonstration of a well-drained cavity with no undrained compartments or loculi.

Key Points

> Success rate of image-guided catheter drainage is 80–90%.
> During transgluteal image-guided drainage, the catheter should be placed close to the sacrum to avoid sciatic nerve injury.
> Deep pelvic abscesses can also be drained using transvaginal or transrectal approaches.
> Percutaneous drainage catheter size is most often 8–14 French.

Suggested Reading

1. Cinat ME, Wilson SE MD, Din AM. Determinants for successful percutaneous image-guided drainage of intra-abdominal abscess. *Arch Surg*. 2002;137:845-849.
2. Jaques P, Mauro M, Safrit H, Yankaskas B, Piggott B. CT features of intraabdominal abscesses: prediction of successful percutaneous drainage. *Am J Roentgenol*. 1986;146:1041-1045.
3. Bakal CW, Sacks D, Burke DR, Cardella JF, Chopra PS, et al. Quality improvement guidelines for adult percutaneous abscess and fluid drainage. *J Vasc Interv Radiol*. 2003;14:S223-S225.
4. Butch RJ, Mueller PR, Ferrucci JT, et al. Drainage of pelvic abscesses through the greater sciatic foramen. *Radiology*. 1986;158:487-491.
5. Hovsepian DM. Transrectal and transvaginal abscess drainage. *J Vasc Interv Radiol*. 1997;8: 501-515.
6. Sperling DC, Needleman L, Eschelman DJ, Hovsepian DM, Lev-Toaff AS. Deep pelvic abscesses: transperineal US-guided drainage. *Radiology*. 1998;208:111-115.

Drainage of Intrathoracic Fluid Collections

Ajay K. Singh

Clinical Features

- Pleural fluid collections are common medical issues, occurring frequently secondary to pneumonia, surgery, infection, and sometimes neoplasm.
- Therapeutic options include thoracentesis, antibiotics, surgical chest tube, or IR catheter drainage and surgery (video-thoracospopic or open decortications). Placing an image-guided percutaneous chest catheter is an attractive alternative to surgically placed chest tubes because of the advantage of precise placement under image guidance and small caliber of the catheter (5–14 F versus approximately 24 F for chest tubes).
- Pleural effuisions resulting primarily from underlying cardiac, liver, or renal conditions are most commonly treated medically and rarely require drainage.

Diagnostic Features

Imaging Appearance

- The US appearance of pleural effusion can be anechoic, complex nonseptated, complex septated, or echogenic (Fig. 1).
- Anechoic collection on US can be transudate or exudate.
- Complex or echogenic collections on US are commonly exudates.
- CT findings of empyema include lenticular shape, split pleura sign, and gas in pleural space.

A.K. Singh
Department of Radiology, Massachusetts General Hospital, Boston, MA, USA

D.A. Gervais and T. Sabharwal (eds.),
Interventional Radiology Procedures in Biopsy and Drainage,
DOI: 10.1007/978-1-84800-899-1_15, © Springer-Verlag London Limited 2011

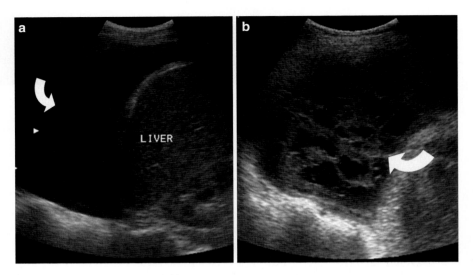

Fig. 1 Ultrasound appearance of right pleural effusion. (**a**) Ultrasound of the right lower chest demonstrates anechoic right-sided pleural effusion (*curved arrow*). Anechoic pleural effusion can be secondary to transudative or exudative fluid. (**b**) Ultrasound of the right lower chest demonstrates complex septated pleural effusion (*curved arrow*). This appearance is typical for exudative pleural effusion or empyema

Thoracentesis

- US or CT guidance is often used for diagnostic and therapeutic thoracentesis (Fig. 2).
- Single thoracentesis along with antibiotic therapy may be effective in the first stage of empyema formation.
- Not effective in definitive management of malignant pleural effusions as majority will recur in 1–3 days. Can be used as temporizing measure.
- It is not as effective in managing parapneumonic effusion because of the need for the high rate of reintervention, especially when the pH of the fluid is low.[1]
- For large volume fluid removal, use small (5–8 F) catheters with direct trocar puncture and connect to vacuum source (bottles or wall suction).

Percutaneous Catheter Drainage

- Typically 5–14 F pigtail drainage catheters are used (Figs. 3–7). Smaller caliber catheters used in pediatric patients and less viscous fluid collections.
- Catheter placed using Trocar or Seldinger's technique.
- Procedure performed under local analgesia. Placement of multiple catheters or difficult placement may require anxiolytics or sedatives.
- Catheter connected to water seal drainage.
- Achieves more than 80% success rate for pleural fluid drainages.

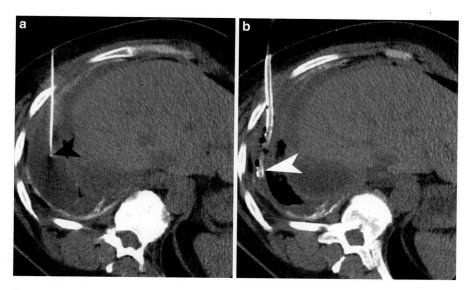

Fig. 2 Catheter drainage of free pleural effusion. (**a**) Intraprocedural noncontrast CT demonstrates an aspiration needle tip (*arrowhead*) placed within a right-sided pleural effusion. High density of the parietal pleura is because of failed pleurodesis in the past. (**b**) Noncontrast CT after aspiration demonstrates a right-sided chest catheter (*arrowhead*) in the pleural space and marked improvement in the right-sided pleural effusion

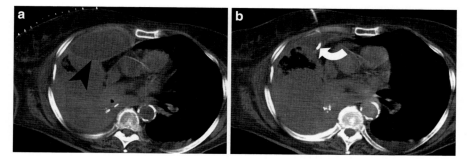

Fig. 3 Catheter drainage of loculated pleural effusion. (**a**) Noncontrast CT of the chest demonstrates a biconvex, lenticular shape loculated pleural fluid collection (*arrowhead*) located anteriorly in the right hemithorax. (**b**) Noncontrast CT of the chest following pigtail catheter (*curved arrow*) drainage demonstrates marked improvement in the size of the pleural fluid collection

Indication for Chest Catheter Drainage

- Pneumothorax
- Empyema
- Malignant pleural effusion
- Traumatic hemopneumothorax
- Postoperative pleural effusions

- Failed surgical chest tube drainage
- Mediastinal and lung abscess

Indicators of Successful Drainage

- Anechoic collection.
- Transudative fluid.
- Lack of septations or multiple loculations.
- Not echogenic.
- No pleural rind.
- However, presence of echoes or loculations does not preclude successful drainage.

Clinical Scenarios

Parapneumonic Effusions and Empyema

- Image-guided catheter drainage usually has success rate of more than 80% and is superior to chest thoracostomy tube drainage because of more precise placement (Figs. 2–3).
- The three stages of empyema are[2]:
  1. *Exudative stage*: The exudative fluid is free flowing and can be managed by drainage with antibiotic therapy.
  2. *Fibrinopurulent stage*: Fluid is more viscous and can be managed with drainage.
  3. *Organizing stage*: Pleural peel formation which requires surgical interventions (open decortication, or video-assisted thoracoscopic surgery).
- Indications for drainage of pleural effusion are based on Light's criteria for exudative effusion, i.e., pH < 7.20, glucose level <60 mg/dL, lactate dehydrogenase level >600 IU/L and presence of bacteria on gram staining.
- Fibrinolytics have been shown to help in drainage by breaking down fibrin products and rendering fluid less viscous.
- One algorithm for finbrinolytics involves 4–6 mg tPA in 25–50 mL 0.9% sterile saline placed into cavity with 30 min dwell time after which drainage is resumed. Repeat twice a day for 3 days and follow-up with chest CT to assess adequacy of response.
- Rapid drainage of large pleural effusion should be controlled to prevent reexpansion edema.
- Catheter removed once there is imaging resolution of empyema and catheter output is less than 20–30 cc/day.

Pneumothorax

- Small bore catheters achieve a high success rate and often used for post-biopsy pneumothorax in radiology department (Figs. 4 and 5).
- Chest drainage catheters are connected to closed underwater seal drainage, which may be connected to a suction pump.

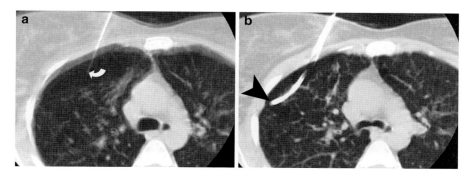

Fig. 4 Pneumothorax treatment using percutaneous image-guided approach. (**a**) Intraprocedural noncontrast chest CT shows a right-sided pneumothorax which is being aspirated with an 18 G needle (*curved arrow*). (**b**) Noncontrast chest CT after placement of a percutaneous chest catheter (*arrowhead*) demonstrating marked improvement in the right-sided pneumothorax

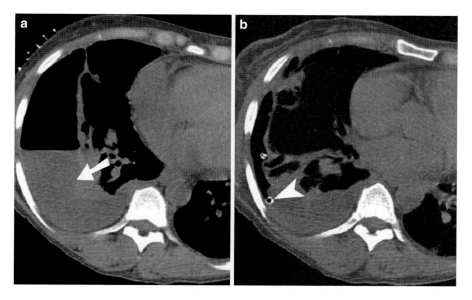

Fig. 5 Percutaneous image-guided treatment of hydropneumothorax. (**a**) Noncontrast chest CT demonstrating a moderately large right hydropneumothorax (*arrow*) with secondary atelectasis in the right lower lobe. (**b**) Noncontrast chest CT after placement of the right chest catheter (*arrowhead*) demonstrating marked improvement in the appearance of the right-sided hydropneumothorax

- Suction pump not routinely used for pneumothorax but has been advocated for nonresolving pneumothorax and after pleurodesis.
- There is no evidence to suggest that clamping of chest drain prior to its removal prevents recurrence of pneumothorax. Clamping of chest catheter followed by a chest x-ray can allow detection of small air leaks, but not routinely recommended.
- Chest catheter removed with patient performing deep expiration or valsalva maneuver.

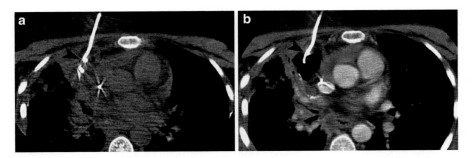

Fig. 6 Lung abscess drainage. (**a**) Noncontrast chest CT scan study demonstrating an 8.5 F pigtail drainage catheter (*arrowhead*) located in an abscess. (**b**) Follow-up chest CT scan study after aspiration with the catheter (*arrowhead*) demonstrates replacement of the fluid in the abscess with air

Lung Abscess

- When nonresponsive to antibiotics, postural drainage and bronchoscopic drainage, image-guided catheter drainage allows high success rate of more than 70% after 10–15 days of drainage.[3]
- If the abscess abuts the pleura, the catheter can be placed without lung parenchymal transgression.
- Typically involves the use of 7–14 F catheter for drainage (Fig. 6).
- Catheter removed once there is imaging resolution of empyema and catheter output is less than 20–30 cc/day.

Mediastinal Abscess

- Although mediastinal infection often require surgical debridgement with drainage, subacute or chronic loculated collection can be managed with percutaneous drainage.
- Precise positioning is more important because of the proximity to major vessels.
- Direct and shortest approach required under CT guidance.
- Drainage reported with 8.3 F or larger caliber pigtail catheter (Fig. 7).

Pleurodesis

- Three tumors most often causing malignant pleural effusion are breast cancer, lung cancer, and lymphoma.
- Imaging-guided catheter drainage and talc sclerotherapy is effective treatment for malignant effusions.

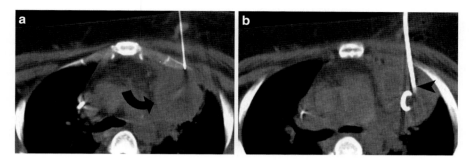

Fig. 7 Mediastinal collection drainage. (**a**) Noncontrast chest CT during the procedure demonstrates a loculated mediastinal fluid collection (*curved arrow*) which is being approached with an 18G aspiration needle. (**b**) Follow-up chest CT during the procedure demonstrates placement of a pigtail drainage catheter (*arrowhead*) into the fluid collection

- Complete regression of pleural effusion achieved in 51–80% and partial resolution in up to 95%.[3]
- The presence of ascites does not adversely affect the overall success of the procedure and should not preclude therapy in such patients.
- Pleural effusions due to malignant tumors recur an average of 4 or 5 days after thoracentesis, so tube thoracostomy, followed by chemical pleurodesis with doxycycline, bleomycin, or talc is useful.
- Implantable pleural catheters such as the Pleurx catheter can induce sufficient pleural irritation by themselves to achieve pleurodesis.

Normal Anatomy

- Each lung enclosed in own pleural space.
- Intercostal vessels vary in location though most commonly closer to bottom of rib than top.
- Internal mammary arteries paramedian.
- Subclavian vessels between clavicle and first rib.

Aberrent/Altered Anatomy

- Post-surgical change may alter anatomy and imaging appearance.
- Single pleural space communicating bilaterally (bovine lung) will predispose to bilateral pneumothorax.
- Avoid chest wall collaterals from venous or arterial obstruction.

Complications

- Hemorrhage.
- Pneumothorax, rare and usually from air introduced during procedure. This will resolve with the catheter in place.
- Lung injury can lead to bleeding into bronchial tree and aspiration into contralateral side. If bleeding appears in endotracheal tube or expectorate, place patient ipsilateral side down. Extremely rare with imaging guidance.

Key Points

> Catheter drainage in the chest is most common in the pleural space.
> Empyemas or other complex effusions typically require an indwelling catheter.
> Fibrinolytics may help drainage when catheter drainage alone is insufficient is spite of satisfactory catheter position.
> Pneumothorax can often be managed with small bore catheters.
> Thoracentesis can be used for acute management, but effusion will usually recur unless underlying cause is addressed
> Pleurodesis has 51–80% success rate in preventing recurrence requiring treatment.
> Lung abscess is typically treated with antibiotics and postural drainage. Catheter drainage may be helpful when these fail.
> A percutaneous tract that avoids lung when entering a lung abscess is ideal to minimize risk of bronchopleural fistula.

Suggested Reading

1. Mitri RK, Brown SD, Zurakowski D, Chung KY, Konez O, et al. Outcomes of primary Image-guided drainage of parapneumonic effusions in children. *Pediatrics*. 2002;110:e37.
2. Light RW. Parapneumonic effusions and empyema. *Clin Chest Med*. 1985;6:55-62.
3. Ghaye B, Dondelinger RF. Image guided thoracic interventions. *Eur Respir J*. 2001;17:507-528.

Liver Cyst / Abscess Drainage

Devrim Akinci

Clinical Features

- Liver cysts can be classified briefly as simple cysts, parasitic (hydatid) cysts, and biliary cystadenomas/cystadenocarcinomas. Cysts can also arise from posttraumatic hematoma.
- Simple cysts can be solitary or multiple. The prevalance has been reported between 2.5% and 7%. Most patients are asymptomatic. Simple cysts can cause symptoms such as abdominal pain, nausea, vomiting, early satiety, and obstructive jaundice.
- Hydatid disease is caused by the larval cestode *Echinococcus granulosus.* It remains endemic in Mediterranean region of Europe, Middle East, South America, Asia, and Africa. Liver is the most frequent site for hydatid disesase.
- Biliary cystadenomas are rare, multilocular cystic tumors of biliary origin.
- Liver abscesses can be classified as pyogenic, amebic, and fungal. They are uncommon, but can be fatal when not diagnosed early and treated promptly. Biliary system disorders and biliary surgery are the most common causes of pyogenic liver abscess. Other facilitating conditions are portal phlebitis, systemic infections through hematogenous dissemination, penetrating trauma, and immunodeficiency due to malignancies, AIDS, and diabetes, etc.
- An amebic abscess results from the infection with the protozoan *Entamoeba hystolytica.*

Diagnostic Evaluation

Laboratory

- In liver abscesses, infected hydatid and simple cysts elevated WBC count is commonly seen.
- Serological tests in diagnosis of hydatid disease are unreliable.

D. Akinci
Radiology Department, Hacettepe University School of Medicine, Ankara, Turkey

D.A. Gervais and T. Sabharwal (eds.),
Interventional Radiology Procedures in Biopsy and Drainage,
DOI: 10.1007/978-1-84800-899-1_16, © Springer-Verlag London Limited 2011

Imaging

- US, CT, and MRI are used in diagnosis of liver cysts and abscesses.
- US is the most useful imaging modality for differentiation of other cystic lesions from hydatid cysts and for classification of hydatid cysts.
- On US simple cysts are anechoic thin-walled structures with acoustic enhancement.
- In Gharbi's classification, the liver hydatid cysts are classified into five groups: type I (pure fluid collection), type II (fluid collection with a split wall), type III (fluid collection with septa), type IV (hydatid cysts with heterogeneous echo patterns), and type V (hydatid cysts with reflecting thick walls).
- WHO classification of US images of hydatid cysts is as follows: CL-cystic lesion: suspicious cystic lesion, CE1: unilocular cyst with uniform anechoic content, CE2: multivesicular, multiseptated cyst, CE3: cyst with detachment of membrane, CE4: cyst with heterogeneous degenerative content, CE5: cyst with calcified wall.
- A simple cyst is seen as a homogeneous and hypoattenuating lesion on unenhanced CT with no enhancement. At MRI, they have low signal intensity on T1W and high signal intensity on T2W images without contrast enhancement.
- Calcification and daughter cysts can be identified at CT in hydatid cysts. MRI demonstrates pericyst as ahypointense rim on both T1W and T2W images.
- Biliary cystadenomas frequently show internal septations, nodularity, focal calcification, surrounding fibrous capsule on US, CT, and MRI. Definitive resection should be the treatment of choice.
- Liver abscesses ususally appear as thick-walled lesions with hypoechogenicity at US, with homogeneous low attenuation at CT, homogeneous low signal intensity on T1W MR images. Enhancing abscess wall on contrast-enhanced CT and MRI can be used to differentiate an abscess from a cystic lesion. Presence of gas can also be detected. An enhancing thick wall and a peripheral zone of edema are common in amebic abscess.

Indications/Contraindications

Simple Cyst

Treatment is indicated if the cysts cause complaints or rapid growth is detected.

Hydatid Cyst

Type I and type II are considered to be most appropriate percutaneous treatment. Type III cysts that do not have nondrainable solid material, some subtypes of type IV that have a significant fluid component, suspected fluid collections after surgical treatment, and infected hydatid cysts are the other indications for percutaneous treatment. The size, number, or location of the hydatid cysts in the liver are not contraindications for percutaneous treatment. The relative contraindications of the treatment of hydatid cysts include some subgroups of type III that contains of nondrainable solid materials and ruptured liver cysts into the biliary system or peritoneum. Treatment is unnecessary in patients with totally calcified liver hydatid cysts (type V) and some subtypes of type IV liver hydatid cysts, which do not contain fluid component.

Liver Abscess

Pyogenic liver abscess is a serious clinical condition with a mortality rate of 6–14%. The current treatment of choice of liver abscess is imaging-guided percutaneous drainage and intravenous antibiotics. Although the initial treatment modality for amebic abscess is medical (metronidazole), percutaneous drainage should be considered for large abscesses with a risk of rupture and for abscesses not responding to medical treatment.

Patient Preparation

- Conscious sedation for percutaneous simple cyst and abscess drainage
- General anesthesia for percutaneous treatment of hydatid cysts due to risk of anaphylaxis

Equipment

- 18–20G Chiba needles
- 6–14 Fr locking pigtail drainage catheters
- Amplatz guide wires
- Hypertonic saline (20–30%) for hydatid cyst treatment
- Sclerosing agent

Pre-proceure Medications

- At least 5 days of oral Albendazole (10 mg/kg/day) treatment prior to percutaneous treatment of hydatid cyst due to risk of spillage during the procedure
- Prophylactic antibiotics for abscess drainage

Procedure

Planning an Access Route

- Avoid vascular and visceral structures during the puncture.
- In percutaneous treatment of hydatid cysts, puncture through the liver parenchyma is preferred in order to eliminate the risk of peritoneal dissemination.

Procedure

- Percutaneous treatment of cysts is performed under US and fluoroscopy guidance.

Simple Cyst

- Aspiration of the cystic fluid and injection of a sclerosing agent is the main principle. Before sclerosing agent installation, cystogram is performed to make sure that there is no biliary communication or peritoneal leakage (Fig. 1). Alcohol is the most commonly used sclerosing agent. Other sclerosing substances such as pantopaque, tetracycline, doxycycline, minocycline chloride, povidone iodine and hypertonic saline have also achieved good results.
- Although single-session sclerotherapy has been proven to be effective, some reports conclude that multiple-session sclerotherapy with prolonged catheterization is more efficient.
- The volume of alcohol injected after aspiration is 30–50% of the cyst volume, the time of exposure is 10–20 min, the maximal dose is 100–200 mL.
- For smaller cysts (<5 cm in diameter), aspiration with an 18G needle followed by sclerotherapy without catheterization is effective.
- For larger cysts, catheterization with 6–8 Fr catheters is performed either with Seldinger or trocar technique. After aspiration and obtaining cystogram, alcohol sclerotherapy is

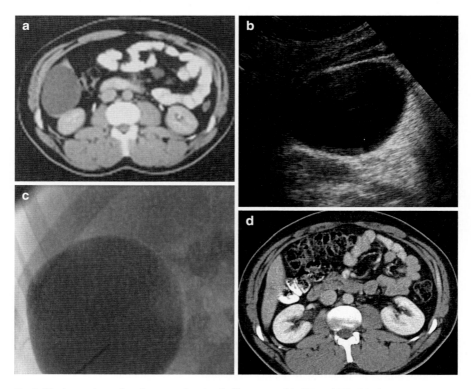

Fig. 1 Single-session sclerotherapy of a simple liver cyst. (**a**) CT and US (**b**) demonstrate 6-cm cyst. After punctue under US guidance cystogram is obtained before sclerotherapy (**c**). In this cyst sclerotherapy was performed with 50 cc of alcohol for 15 minutes. At CT, obtained 1 year after the procedure, no cyst was detected (**d**)

done and the cyst is evacuated. For single session the catheter is removed, however, if multiple session is planned, sclerotherapy sessions are repeated every day until the drainage stops.

Hydatid Cyst

- Three different techniques are used for percutaneous treatment of liver hydatid cysts. PAIR technique (**P**uncture, **A**spiration of cyst content, **I**njection of hypertonic saline solution, and **R**easpiration of all fluid), catheterization technique, and modified catheterization techniques.
- In PAIR and catheterization, hypertonic saline (20–30%) is used to irrigate and inactivate the cyst. This should remain in the cavity for approximately 10 min in order to destroy all the viable protoscolices (Fig. 2).
- The cyst is punctured under US guidance and obtaining clear crystal fluid is characteristic. After puncture and aspiration, before hypertonic injection cystogram is obtained to ensure that there is no biliary communication. If there is no communication, hypertonic saline is injected. After injection, detachment of germinative membrane can be detected with US.
- In catheterization a 6–10 Fr catheter is placed by Seldinger technique after the first three steps of PAIR and reaspiration is performed through the catheter. This not only makes the procedure easier for cysts larger than 6 cm in diameter (volume > ~100 cc), but also allows safe sclerotherapy using alcohol if desired before the catheter removal.
- Modified catheterization technique is used for the complicated cases such as some subgroups of type III that contain nondrainable solid material. In this technique, a 14–16 Fr catheter is inserted into the cavity whose nondrainable content is also evacuated besides the cystic component via the catheter with irrigation.

Liver Abscess

- Most of the liver abscesses can be drained by using US with or without fluoroscopy as imaging guidance. However, for some abscesses with deep location or air content, which cannot be seen with US, CT guidance is needed.
- Since it is not always possible to diagnose fluid collection with imaging alone, diagnostic aspiration is required. If infected fluid is aspirated catheter (8–14 Fr locking pigtail) is placed either with Seldinger or tandem trocar technique (Fig. 3).
- Although the catheter drainage is more effective, percutaneous needle aspiration can also be used for abscesses smaller than 5 cm in diameter. However, this needle aspiration technique requires careful follow-up, since repeated aspirations might be needed.

Immediate Post-proceure Care

- Samples are sent for biochemical, cytological, and bacteriological examinations.
- Bed rest for 4 h and check vital signs.

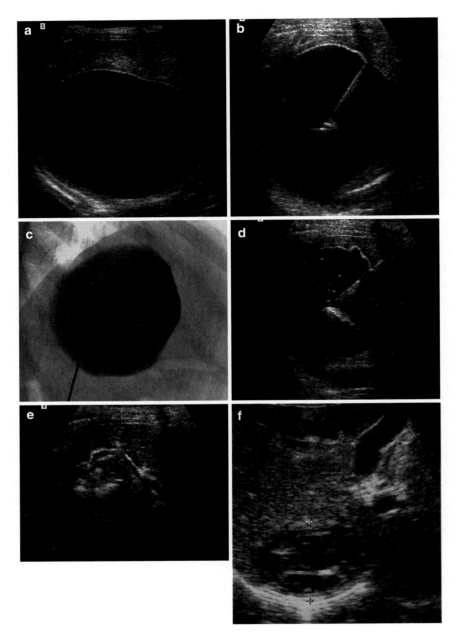

Fig. 2 Percutaneous treatment of hydatid cyst with PAIR. (**a**) US shows type 1 liver hydatid cyst. After puncture (**b**) under US guidance with an 18 G Chiba needle and aspiration of the cyst fluid, cystogram (**c**) is obtained before injecting hypertonic saline (**d**). All the cyst content is reaspirated (**e**) approximately 10 minutes after hypertonic saline injection. One year after the treatment US shows size reduction and disappearance of fluid component (**f**)

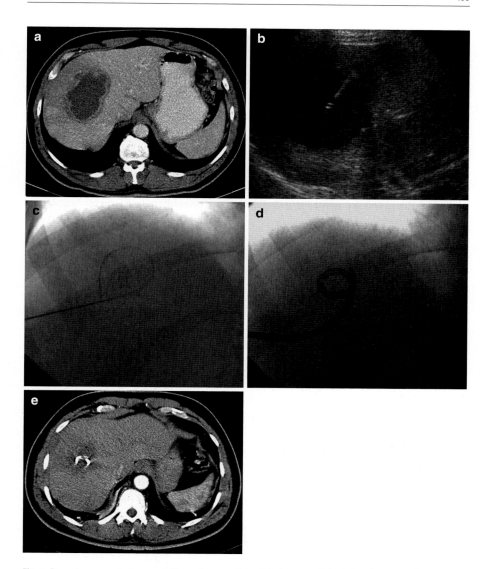

Fig. 3 Percutaneous drainage of liver abscess. (**a**). CT shows a right lobe abscess. Abscess was punctured with an 18 G Chiba needle under US guidance (**b**). After aspiration of purulent fluid, a 10 Fr drainage catheter was placed with Seldinger technique (**c** and **d**). (**e**). 10 days after catheterization, CT demonstrates no abscess cavity and the catheter is in place

- Simple cysts can be managed in outpatient basis.
- Percutaneous hydatid cyst treatment and percutaneous abscess drainage procedures are performed in inpatient basis.

- After placement of a percutaneous draiange catheter in a liver abscess, excessive manipulation, overdistension by injecting saline, or contrast should be avoided because of the risk of postprocedure sepsis.
- Patients should undergo clinical follow-up and daily rounds until they are discharged.

Follow-up and Postprocedure Medications

Simple cyst

If the catheter is left for multisession sclerotherapy, sclerotherapy is repeated everyday. When the daily drainage is less than 10 cc/24 h, catheter is removed.

Hydatid cyst

Oral Albendazole treatment is continued for a month. If catheterization technique is performed, the catheter is left until the daily drainage is less than 10 cc/24 h. Before removal sclerotherapy with alcohol is performed unless the fluid is bilious. If the amount of bilious drainage is high, ERCP for papillotomy should be considered.

Ultrasonography is performed once in every 3 months during the first year after the procedure and then twice a year at the second year and once for the following years.

Liver abscess

The clinical status of the patient, daily amount of drainage, catheter patency, catheter position, and catheter site should be inspected. If clinical (pain, fever), laboratory (leukocyte count and sedimentation rate), and radiological improvement (loss or reduction of cavity, the amount of daily drainage not more than 10 mL/24 h) exist, the catheter is withdrawn.

Results

Simple Cyst

Percutaneous aspiration without sclerotherapy is associated with high recurrence rates (78–100%). The average volume reduction after single-session alcohol sclerotherapy exceeds 90%. For larger cysts multiple-sclerotherapy sessions have been proposed. Recurrence rates around 20% have been reported after single-session sclerotherapy.

Hydatid Cyst

The success rate of percutaneous hydatid cysts is between 90% and 100% in large series. The recurrence rate is less than 4%. Recurrent cysts can also be treated percutaneously.

Liver Abscess

The success rate of percutaneous drainage of liver abscess is over 90%. Recurrence rates have been reported to be around 10%.

Alternative Therapies

- Surgical approaches for simple cysts are open or laparoscopic unroofing, drainage, and hepatic resection.
- Surgical interventions for hydatid cysts consist of both conservative and radical approaches. Conservative techniques are simple tube drainage, marsupialization, capitonnage, deroofing, and cystectomy, with or without omentoplasty. Radical procedures include total pericystectomy, partial hepatectomy, and lobectomy.
- For patients with pyogenic liver abscess, surgical treatment is occasionally required when percutaneous drainage fails.

Complications

Simple Cyst

Overall complication rates are reported to be less than 10%. Complications such as pain during sclerotherapy, bleeding, cyst infection, pleural effusion can develope.

Hydatid Cyst

Death due to anaphylactic shock was reported in two cases (0.1–0.2%). Minor complications are some allergic reactions such as urticaria, itching, and hypotension that may be treated by antihistaminics and fever not more than 38.5°C, which does not require any medication. Other minor complications (10%) are infection in the cavity, fistula between cavity and the biliary system.

Liver Abscess

Overall complication rates are reported to be less than 15%. The major complications include hemorrhage, sepsis, and pleural complications such as pneomothorax, hemothorax, and empyema. Minor complications include local pain and bleeding, and catheter-related complications such as blockage, kink, dislodgement, and catheter site infection.

Key Points

> Preprocedural imaging is critical in differential diagnosis of cystic lesions and classification of hydatid cysts (US findings), which is important for planning the treatment.
> Before sclerosing agent installation, any fistula or leak should be eliminated with cystogram.
> General anesthesia is preferred in percutaneous hydatid cyst treatment due to risk of anaphylaxis.
> After percutaneous liver abscess drainage excessive manipulation and overdistension should be avoided because of the risk of postprocedure sepsis.

Suggested Reading

1. Akhan O, Ozmen MN. Percutaneous treatment of liver hydatid cysts. *Eur J Radiol*. 1999;32: 76-85.
2. Akinci D, Akhan O, Ozmen MN, et al. Percutaneous drainage of 300 intraabdominal abscesses with long term follow-up. *Cardiovasc Interv Radiol*. 2005;28:744-750.
3. Rajak CL, Gupta S, Jain S, et al. Percutaneous treatment of liver abscesses: needle aspiration versus catheter drainage. *Am J Roentgenol*. 1998;170:1035-1039.
4. van Sonnenberg E, Wroblicka JT, D'agostino HB, et al. Symptomatic hepatic cysts: percutaneous drainage and sclerosis. *Radiology*. 1994;190:387-392.
5. World Health Organization. PAIR: punture, aspiration, injection, re-aspiration. An option for the treatment of Cystic Echinococcosis. http://libdoc.who.int/hq/2001/WHO_CDS_CSR_APH_2001.6

Drainage of Pancreatic Abscess and Fluid Collections

Nicos I. Fotiadis

Clinical-Pathologic Features

Pancreatic fluid collections represent a diverse group of lesions of various causes, severity, and treatments. Most common *causes* include acute and chronic pancreatitis and less commonly pancreatic trauma and collections post-pancreatic surgery.

Based on their pathologic changes and the imaging findings pancreatic fluid collections are divided into four types (Atlanta classification).

- *Acute fluid collections* occur early in the course of acute pancreatitis and lack a wall of fibrous or granulation tissue. The majority resolves spontaneously and do not need intervention. The collections, which persist for 4–6 weeks will progress to become pseudocysts and if infected abscesses.
- *Pseudocyst* is a collection of pancreatic juice enclosed by a wall of fibrous and granulation tissue.
- *Pancreatic necrosis* is a focal or diffuse area of nonviable pancreatic parenchyma that is usually associated with peripancreatic fat necrosis.
- *Pancreatic abscess* is a circumscribed collection of pus typically in proximity to the pancreas containing little or no pancreatic necrosis. Pancreatic abscesses include infected pseudocysts, late infected fluid collections, and postoperative collections.

Imaging

- Contrast-enhanced *CT* is the examination of choice. It delineates the areas of pancreatic necrosis, the size and extent of the collections, and reveals life-threatening pseuodoaneurysm.
- Ultrasound (US) is usually of limited value due to overlying bowel.

N.I. Fotiadis
Radiology Department, Barts and The London NHS Trust, London, UK

D.A. Gervais and T. Sabharwal (eds.),
Interventional Radiology Procedures in Biopsy and Drainage,
DOI: 10.1007/978-1-84800-899-1_17, © Springer-Verlag London Limited 2011

- Endoscopic ultrasound (EUS) with FNA is extremely useful in the differential diagnosis of a pseudocyst from a cystic neoplasm.
- MRI and MRCP are not well suited in the acute setting. These offer invaluable information in chronic pancreatitis defining the anatomy of the biliary tree and the pancreatic duct, revealing strictures, stones, and tumors.
- Endoscopic retrograde cholangiopancreatography (ERCP) is used if endoscopic sphincterotomy or pancreatic stenting is contemplated.

Indications/Contraindications

Acute fluid collections do not usually need any intervention as many resolve in 4–6 weeks.

Pseudocysts

- Asymptomatic <5 cm pseudocysts should be monitored likely to resolve spontaneously.
- Intervention is indicated for the following:
  — Symptomatic pseudocysts causing pain
  — Suspected infection
  — Persistence of a large (>5 cm) pseudocyst
  — Increasing size of the pseudocyst
  — Biliary or gastrointestinal obstruction

Pancreatic Necrosis

- Drainage of sterile necrosis is not indicated.
- Infected necrosis needs aggressive drainage with multiple large bore catheters in close collaboration with the surgeons for surgical, laparoscopic or percutaneous necrosectomy.

Pancreatic Abscess

Absolute indication for percutaneous drainage (Figs. 1 and 2).

Image Guidance-Access Route

- CT is the preferred imaging modality for guiding percutaneous pancreatic drainages.
- Ultrasound can be used for drainage of large pseudocysts or collections near the anterolateral abdominal wall.

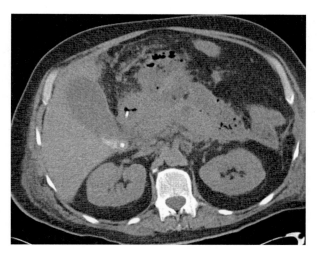

Fig. 1 Large pancreatic abscess at the pancreatic bed and the left anterior pararenal space in a patient with severe sepsis

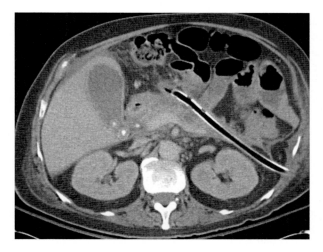

Fig. 2 Computed tomography (CT) scan 12 weeks postdrainage with a large 28F multihole catheter, inserted through a retroperitoneal approach. Complete resolution of the collection

Access routes are chosen to avoid traversing intestine and contaminating potentially sterile collection.

- For collections in or near the pancreatic tail the most commonly used route is through the left anterior pararenal space.
- For collections in or near the pancreatic head, body and the lesser sac access through the gastrocolic ligament is usually obtained.
- Main advantage of the transgastric approach is that there is no formation of persistent pancreato-cutaneous fistula. It can also be used for percutaneous cystgastrostomy.

Technique

- Fine needle (22G Chiba-15 cm long) aspiration for bacteriology should be performed to differentiate between sterile and infected pancreatic necrosis in patients with sepsis syndrome.
- CT guidance is mandatory to avoid bowel contamination of necrosis.
- If nothing could be aspirated inject 2–3 mL of sterile saline and aspirate back.
- Strict sterility is imperative. Samples from at least two areas should be taken.

Pancreatic Abscess-Infected Necrosis

- Procedure performed under CT guidance. Use an 18–19G long two part needle. Seldinger technique is easier to master from the inexperience operator than the Trocar.
- Use a short (80 cm) extra stiff Amplatz wire. Making a larger curve at the distal end of the wire will facilitate coiling of the wire in the abscess cavity.
- For difficult access and less experience operators the Neff or Accustic set (22G needle/0.018 in. wire) could be used.
- Generous amount of local anesthetic with conscious sedation or general anesthesia in some cases. Fairly large skin incision would help insertion of a large bore catheter.
- Perform serial dilatation.
- Depending on the viscosity of the collection large bore catheters are needed, ranging from 14 to 28F.
- For loculated noncommunicating collections more than one catheters are needed.

Pseudocysts

- Smaller locking pigtail catheters (8–12F) will suffice for drainage of most pseudocysts.
- Transgastric approach – if possible – is the preferred access. Prevents the formation of pancreaticocutaneous fistula.
- Drainage duration will depend on whether the pseudocyst communicates with the pancreatic duct.
    — Communication with a normal pancreatic duct without downstream obstruction may take 4–6 weeks of catheter drainage but is likely to be successful.
    — Communication with an obstructed downstream pancreatic duct makes catheter drainage highly unlikely to succeed and surgery should be considered.
- Clamp the drainage catheter for 24 h before catheter removal to ensure that pseudocyst does not recur.
- Internal stent-assisted cystgastrostomy can also be performed if there is close apposition of the pseudocyst to the posterior wall of the stomach.

- Initial puncture is made with a one stick-needle system under CT guidance traversing the stomach.
- Patient is brought to fluoroscopy and a 12 Fr sheath is placed into the pseudocyst using lateral fluoroscopy.
- The stomach is distended with air via an N/G tube.
- A 10 or 12 Fr plastic stent is placed between the stomach and the pseudocyst.
- The stent is removed after 3–4 months endoscopically.
- Octreotide acetate (Sandostatin, Biochemie, Schaftenau, Austria) is indicated for prolonged drainage, high-output drainage, pseudocyst recurrence, or pancreatic fistula.

Aftercare

- Pancreatic drainage can last for weeks making catheter care of paramount importance. Inspect catheter entry site for signs of infection and evaluate catheter output.
- Irrigation with saline three or more times a day until the returning fluid is clear. The technique includes first aspiration of all the fluids that could be withdrawn, followed by gentle instillation of 20 mL aliquots of saline. Aspirate and discard the fluid. Repeat until the returning fluid is reasonably clear.
- Frequent follow-up with CT is helpful to check for residual and/or undrained pockets. The interventional radiologist, who perform the procedure should interpret the CT scan and adjust further management, which includes repositioning or upsizing the catheter and insertion of further drain.

Endpoint

- End point for catheter removal include no further drainage, no evidence of fistula, and no recurrence noted at follow-up imaging after the catheter has been clamped for 2–3 days.

Alternative Therapies

For pseudocysts:

- Endoscopic cystgastrostomy or transpapillary stenting when there is communication of the cyst with the pancreatic duct.
- Surgical cystgastrostomy or cyst removal.

For pancreatic necrosis:
- Surgical debridement/necrosectomy when percutaneous options are exhausted.

Key Points

> Contrast-enhanced CT for diagnosis, planning and guidance of the procedure.
> Exclude the presence of a pseudoaneurysm, and a cystic pancreatic tumor.
> For pancreatic abscesses use large bore (20–28F) multihole catheters.
> Long-term drainage with close follow-up of the patient and close cooperation and communication with the surgeon and gastroenterologist is the key for success.

Suggested Reading

1. Aghdassi A, Mayerle J, Kraft M, et al. Diagnosis and treatment of pancreatic pseudocyst in chronic pancreatitis. *Pancreas*. 2008;36:105-112.
2. Lee MJ, Wittich GR, Mueller PR. Percutaneous intervention in acute pancreatitis. *Radiographics*. 1998;18:711-724.
3. Neff R. Pancreatic pseudocysts and fluid collections: percutaneous approaches. *Surg Clin North Am*. 2001;81(2):399-403.
4. Shankar S, van Sonnenberg E, Silverman SG, Tuncali K, Banks PA. Imaging and percutaneous management of acute complicated pancreatitis. *Cardiovasc Intervent Radiol*. 2004;27: 567-580.

Percutaneous Biliary Drainage and Stenting

Adam A. Hatzidakis

Clinical Features

Percutaneous transhepatic biliary drainage (PTBD) is a therapeutic procedure, which leads to the percutaneous drainage of the obstructed bile duct system.

The underlying disease is either malignancy of the bile ducts itself, or of adjacent organs or structures such as pancreas, lymphnodes, the gallbladder, or the stomach.

PTBD is also performed in benign conditions due to biliary stones or strictures, post-transplantation strictures, and after surgery (iatrogenic injuries).

Diagnostic Evaluation

Clinical

- Check for patient's history of medication, and all previously undertaken operations of the upper abdomen, especially affecting the hepatobiliary area.
- Ascites

Laboratory

- Full blood count, coagulation, hepatic and renal studies. Any imbalances should be corrected before the procedure.

A.A. Hatzidakis
Medical School of Heraklion, University of Crete, Crete, Greece

D.A. Gervais and T. Sabharwal (eds.),
Interventional Radiology Procedures in Biopsy and Drainage,
DOI: 10.1007/978-1-84800-899-1_18, © Springer-Verlag London Limited 2011

Imaging

- Pre-interventional multimodality imaging is imperative for defining the cause of the obstruction.
- The level of an associated stricture can usually be found with a simple ultrasound examination (US) of the region. US can also depict the presence of an obstructing mass, the dilated biliary system, lymph node enlargement, a hydropic gallbladder, free intraperitoneal fluid, possible vascular disorders, lobar liver atrophy, or the presence of hypervascular intrahepatic masses, i.e., hemangiomas or metastases.
- Coronal reconstruction of the CT-image corresponds the anterior-posterior fluroscopy projection and can be very helpful to better understand the anatomic background.
- High-quality multiplanar MRI combined with MRCP images provides the best information about the cause and level of obstruction. MRCP offers additional information about biliary anatomy and possible variations, GB position, presence of ascites, liver size, and colon interposition.

Indications

- Obstructive jaundice with bilirubin elevation/sepsis and ERCP failure
- ERCP not possible, e.g., previous gastric surgery
- Inoperable patient

Alternative Therapies

- ERCP and plastic or metallic stent placement
- Open or laparoscopic surgery

Contraindications

- Massive ascites
- Incorrectable coagulopathy
- Uncooperative patient
- Progressive hepatic failure

Specific Complications

If the site of obstruction is in the distal CBD, and the patient has an incorrectable coagulopathy, or no safe hepatic access, a percutaneous cholecystostomy can be performed instead.

Patient Preparation

- Antibiotic prophylaxis is advisable before any biliary procedure. A combination of Gentamycin, Ampicillin, and Metronidaziole can be used as combination therapy or Tazocin (tazobactam/piperacillin) can be used as a solitary agent
- Infectious conditions, such as cholangitis, cholecystitis, pancreatitis, or sepsis, must be treated with IV administration of antibiotic drugs before drainage.
- It is also advisable to start patients on IV fluids before PTBD because they are almost always dehydrated and at risk for post-procedure hepatorenal failure

Anatomy

Normal Anatomy

- Right anterior and posterior sectoral ducts join to form the right main biliary duct.
- Left lobe segment 2 and 3 ducts join to form the left main biliary duct.
- Right and left main biliary ducts join to form the common hepatic duct.
- Common hepatic duct and cystic duct join to form the common bile duct (CBD).

Aberrant Anatomy

- Right anterior or posterior sectoral ducts join the left segment 2 or 3 duct or the left main bile duct.
- Left lobe ducts joining a right lobe duct or the right main bile duct.
- Right lobe aberrant ducts join the common hepatic duct.
- Cystic duct joins the common hepatic duct very low just above the papilla of Vater.

Equipment

- Fluoroscopic x-ray equipment with Ultrasound
- Catheters/Needles
  - Fine 21G Chiba needle for initial biliary puncture.
  - An 18G needle with plastic coverage for second puncture or one stick needle system with 0.018 in. guide wire and 4 Fr sheath (e.g., Neff set, Cook, Bjaerskov, Denmark).
  - Hydrophilic 0.035 in. curved guide wire for crossing the obstruction.
  - Extra stiff 0.035 in. guide wire exchanged after the papilla of Vater is crossed.
  - 8 Fr self-locking drainage catheter for external drainage.
  - 8 Fr self-locking biliary drainage catheter for internal–external drainage.
  - A 10-mm wide metallic stent carried over a 6 Fr catheter.

Pre/Peri-procedure Medications

- Adequate conscious sedation and analgesia is mandatory, because the PTBD can be very painful. In fact, some interventionalists perform PTBD under GA.
- IV fluids should be continued during drainage, as a prophylactic measure against hepatorenal failure.

Procedure

- Percutaneous transhepatic cholangiography (PTC) is the basic procedure for opacification of dilated biliary tree. It is performed under sterile conditions, with the patient in supine position. After percutaneous local anesthesia, liver is punctured duct is punctured with a fine 21–22G Chiba needle, under fluoroscopic guidance and/or ultrasound. Enter the liver in the right middle axillary line between the 9th and 11th intercostal space targeting the xiphoid, keeping the needle on a horizontal level until reaching the level of the right lateral spine margin. For the left biliary duct system, puncture the anterior abdominal wall just under the xiphoid/left costochondral junction, aiming posterior and to the right, ideally under US guidance.

Planning an Access Route

- Depending on the site of obstruction, the presence of liver atrophy or ascites, a left lobe puncture instead of the right may be decided. The presence of liver metastases or hemangiomas may alter the puncture site as well, or even make the use of real-time US guidance necessary for the initial puncture (Fig. 1).
- After opacification of the obstructed biliary system, decision must be made about the site of puncture for introduction of the drainage catheter. A bile duct, as peripheral as possible should be chosen (Fig. 2).
- In some cases, when dealing with patients with several intrahepatic stones proximal to a benign stricture, access may need to be modified by choosing a particular bile duct for the initial drainage, to provide the best access for the subsequent lithotripsy.
- For common bile duct (CBD) lesions, right-sided approach is preferred, except in cases of ascites or colon interposition. Right-sided route provides a straighter access for catheter and guide-wire manipulation and keeps the operator's hands out of the x-ray beam.
- Hilar lesions deserve special mention. These lesions are classified according to the Bismuth classification. If patients are nonsurgical candidates, Bismuth stages 2 and 3 are best palliated by PTBD and stenting. ERCP and stenting or PTBD can be used for stage 1, if surgery is not possible. Palliation of patients with stage 4 disease is difficult with any technique, but percutaneous approach is usually preferred.

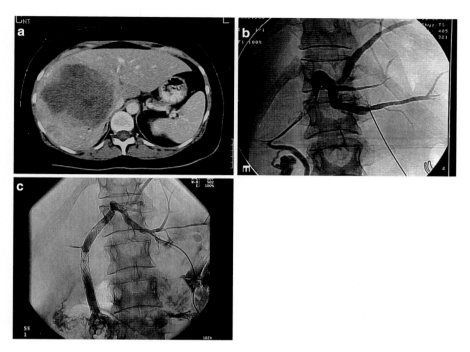

Fig. 1 (**a**) Computed tomography (CT) scan with a large liver tumor in a jaundiced patient. (**b**) Only a peripheral left liver puncture can be performed with safety. (**c**) Metallic stent in situ

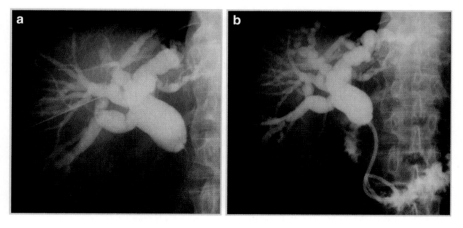

Fig. 2 (**a**) Initial puncture is performed through a dilated seventh segment bile duct. (**b**) Drainage catheter placement is performed after a more peripheral puncture of a sixth segment bile duct

- With hilar obstructions, careful evaluation of pre-procedure MRCP imaging is vital. Anatomical variations should be checked. If the right anterior or posterior sectoral ducts drain to the left main duct, then left lobe drainage may be sufficient for palliation. If the tumor is mainly involving the left ducts, then draining the right may be the best approach and vice versa. However, if draining is in only the left lobe, the left lobe should be of sufficient size to provide palliation. There is little point in draining a small left liver lobe as it will not provide relief for jaundice or pruritus. Additionally, hilar tumors tend to grow proximally along the biliary ducts so that puncturing a peripheral duct for access is vital if stenting. You ideally need 2–3 cm of stent above the obstruction for good palliation.

Performing the Procedure

Technique

There are two major techniques for introduction of a biliary catheter:

- The fine 21–22G needle technique
- The 18G needle technique
- Advantage of the fine-needle technique is that even multiple needle passages may not cause complications, so the procedure can be considered safer than using the 18G needle. However, the fine-needle technique might be difficult in inexperienced hands.
- PTC is performed initially as described above. Entry into a bile duct recognized by injection of diluted contrast material (CM) through the Chiba needle. CM injected into hepatic or portal veins flows away from the needle tip reasonably smartly. CM in the bile duct flows slowly away like wax flowing down a candle.
- When access to the bile duct is gained, a diagnostic cholangiogram is performed. If the duct that has been entered is appropriate for drainage access, then the 0.018-in. guidewire is manipulated through the Chiba needle into the bile duct. If the bile duct is not suitable, the Chiba needle is left in place and another Chiba needle is used to access a more favorable duct.
- The 4 Fr sheath system that is part of the one stick system is then tracked via the 0.018-in. guidewire. Remember to unhook the stiffener form the sheath when the duct is reached. The stiffener will not travel well through any bends. The 0.018-in. guidewire and inner plastic stylet are then removed and an 0.035-in. J-guide wire is inserted.
- A 40-cm hockey stick catheter is placed over the 0.035-in. guide wire and CM is injected to outline the exact level of the obstruction and to see if there is a nipple to suggest the course of the obstructed bile duct. A 0.035-in. Terumo guide wire is used to negotiate the obstructed segment and manipulated into the duodenum to the level of the ligament of Treitz. The Terumo guide wire is then exchanged for a superstiff guide wire.
- The percutaneous track is then dilated with 7 and 9 Fr dilators and the 8 Fr multi-sidehole pigtail catheter is placed. Note that placing a 9 Fr peel-away sheath may aid catheter placement.

- CM is injected to make sure that there are sideholes above and below the obstruction and the catheter secured.
- The only difference using the 18G needle technique is that after initial PTC, an appropriate peripheral biliary duct is chosen for puncturing with an 18G Chiba needle. Through this needle, a 0.035-in. Terumo guide wire is negotiated through the stricture, following tract dilatation and catheter placement as described above.

If opacification of multiple obstructed bile ducts occurs, the operator should try to drain as many opacified ducts as possible in order to avoid bacterial contamination and post-procedural cholangitis.

The drainage of the bile ducts is performed with a multi-sidehole pigtail catheter. The catheter is placed internally across the narrowed duct, having the external end connected to a drainage bag. The catheter is secured to the skin with sutures. Self-locking catheters are preferred in order to minimize the dislocation risk.

Endpoint

- The percutaneous catheter is placed across the stenosed/obstructed CBD, so that bile is draining through the catheter toward the bowel loops (sideholes proximal and distal to stricture).
- The drainage procedure can be extended with the placement of a permanent metallic stent, which keeps the stenosed biliary duct patent, without the need for a catheter (Fig. 1c). Metallic biliary stents have been shown to provide the best palliative treatment for non-resectable malignant obstructive jaundice, allowing longer patency rates than plastic endoprostheses. If initial transhepatic drainage is completed without causing any significant complications, especially bleeding, primary metallic stenting can follow as a single-step procedure.

The keys for shortening the total intervention time are the following:

— Careful initial transhepatic drainage, to allow primary metallic stenting, in the absence of hemobilia.
— Immediate optimal stent expansion, so that free bile drainage is guaranteed and the possibility of cholangitis decreases.
— Placement of a thin 4–5 Fr catheter after stent placement, which can be removed 1 or 2 days post-procedure.

Immediate Post-procedure Care

- The whole procedure may last 1–2 h, depending on the grade of difficulty and the cooperation of the patient.
- Catheter must be carefully fixed on the skin.
- Monitor for bleeding complications and hepatorenal syndrome.

Follow-up and Post-procedure Medications

- In general, the patient is kept in the Hospital until recovery. Usually the main post-procedural complaint is pain, especially if drainage is placed intercostally. Appropriate pain medication, which may include opiates, may be necessary.
- Blood pressure and pulse must be monitored, hematocrit must be measured, and catheter site must be checked frequently.
- Patient can eat and drink normally.
- Patient must be careful not to dislodge the catheter.
- The catheter skin entrance site must be cleaned and sterilized every 1–2 days.
- The drainage catheter should be flushed with 10-mL saline preferably every 8 h.
- At the time of catheter removal the percutaneous tract can be plugged with gelfoam pledgets delivered through a peel-away sheath. This greatly diminishes post-catheter removal pain and bile leak. Another option is to fill the catheter tract with tissue-glue (mixed with lipiodol) while slowly removing a 4–5 Fr catheter from the liver.

Results

Technical success of the percutaneous biliary drainage depends on the experience of the interventional radiologist performing the drainage. It can be as high as nearly 100%. Clinical efficacy is usually lower but still over 90%.

If metallic stenting is also performed, stent patency is an important issue. Patency depends on the cause and the site of the stenosis, but can reach 6–12 months or more.

Metallic Stenting

- Stents are used as a more permanent palliative treatment option. Initially plastic endoscopically inserted stents of 8–12 Fr size were used. Their main problems were a 30-day mortality rate of 15–24%, migration, early occlusion usually after 2–3 months, and infection. Thus, metallic stents were developed in order to overcome these complications.
- It is now proven that metallic stents offer a 30-day mortality rate of only 5%, longer patency of about 5–6 months, providing better bile flow through an 8–10-mm wide lumen and have a lower reintervention rate. Endoscopic and percutaneous placement is possible. The latter is preferred in cases of hilar tumors or if endoscopy fails.
- Technically, percutaneous metallic stenting is a relative easy procedure after internal drainage has succeeded. The stents have a delivery system of 6 Fr size, minimizing liver parenchyma damage, and enabling primary stenting more safely.

- After careful measurement of stricture length, a stent of at least 3–4 cm extra length must be chosen, so that proximal and distal overstenting with 1–2 cm in each side is possible. In this way tumor overgrowth can be avoided (proximal part) and the papilla can be kept open for better bile drainage (distal part).
- Nevertheless, stent occlusion still remains a problem due to sludge incrustation or tumoral ingrowth and overgrowth. Covered stents have been developed to overcome these complications. Nowadays, covered stents with ePTFE coverage have been clinically tried in comparison to the uncovered stents, showing relative good results regarding prevention of tumor ingrowth. Stent dysfunction tends to be significantly lower for covered stents ($P=0.046$), while tumor ingrowth occurred exclusively in bare stent. Stent migration is prohibited by side-anchoring fins. Despite the relative large stent carrying catheter size of 10 Fr, no significant difference of complication rate is noticed in relation to uncovered stents with delivery system of 6 Fr size.

Complications

Biliary drainage and metallic stenting is safe, with acceptable complication rates (10–15% minor, 4–5% major) and low procedure-related mortality between 0.8% and 3.4%. Procedure-related complications like stent misplacement or occlusion can be corrected by placement of a second stent. Severe bleeding is uncommon and should be treated conservatively with blood transfusions, or if bleeding persists, by means of arterial embolization.

- If there is significant hemobilia, check that the side holes of catheter have not migrated back to lie across a portal or hepatic vein. If this is the case the catheter needs to be advanced.
- If bleeding persists, the catheter can be upsized to tamponade the bleeding site.
- For persistent bleeding, transarterial embolization should be performed

How to Avoid Complications

Make sure that the patient receives antibiotic prophylaxis and IV fluids pre-procedure. If the patient is septic at the time of PTBD, the minimum needed to provide drainage should be performed. Do not inject too much CM and place a small pigtail catheter above the obstruction. Careful, peripheral transhepatic drainage, to allow primary metallic stenting, in the absence of hemobilia. Immediate optimal stent expansion, if necessary with the help of balloon dilatation through a 6 Fr sheath, so that free bile drainage is guarantied and possibility of cholangitis minimizes. Placement of a thin 4–5 Fr safety catheter after stent placement, which can be retrieved 1–2 days later.

Medication

Percutaneous biliary drainage is often painful. Drug therapy is aimed toward prevention and management of complications like pain, infection, or nausea.

- *Pain control*: prophylactic anti-inflammatory strong analgesia is often needed and should be given early. Patient-controlled analgesia should be established.
- *Infection control:* broad-spectrum antibiotics are recommended as transductal bacterial colonization is possible.
- *Sickness control:* antiemetics should be given.
- *Hydration*: intravenous normal saline.

Follow-up

- Biochemical tests for following bilirubin and hepatic enzymes level.
- Ultrasonographic control for imaging of biliary tree decompression.
- Cholangiographic control through the drainage catheter to check correct stent placement and expansion.

Key Points

> Review the pre-procedural imaging and plan the procedure
> Ensure that you understand the rationale for treating each patient. This will enable:
>   - Correct choice of percutaneous puncture site
>   - Correct choice of bile duct puncture for drainage placement
>   - Avoid manipulation, which might increase the complication risk
>   - Consider the possibility of immediate metallic stent placement
> Ensure adequate supportive therapy before, during, and after the procedure.
> Never start percutaneous puncture until you have personally reviewed the imaging and the bleeding parameters.
> *Stop if uncertain, especially if there is risk of arterial damage or intraperitoneal hemorrhage.*

Suggested Reading

1. Rossi P, ed. *Biliary Tract Radiology*. Berlin/Heidelberg/New York: Springer-Verlag; 1997.
2. Mueller P (ed), Venbrux AC (guest editor). Biliary intervention procedures. Semin Interv Radiol. 1996;13(3).
3. Burhenne HJ, guest editor. Interventional Radiology of the Biliary Tract, The Radiological Clinics of North America. W.B. Saunders, Philadelphia, PA; 1990.

4. Lammer J. Biliary endoprostheses. Plastic versus metal stents. *Radiol Clin North Am.* 1990;28(6):1211-1222.
5. Krokidis M, Fanelli F, Orgera G, Bezzi M, Passariello R, Hatzidakis A. Percutaneous treatment of malignant jaundice due to extrahepatic cholangiocarcinoma: covered viabil stent versus uncovered wallstents. *Cardiovasc Intervent Radiol.* 2009;32:647-657.

Percutaneous Cholecystostomy and Cholecystolithotomy

Manpreet S. Gulati

Percutaneous Cholecystostomy

Introduction

Acute cholecystitis is a relatively common condition with high associated risk of morbidity and mortality. Symptomatic calculus cholecystitis generally requires treatment by early cholecystectomy under antibiotic prophylaxis and has been shown to be superior to delayed surgery in several prospective trials. Mortality can be as low as 0.5% in younger age groups, but in the elderly and critically ill, mortality can be higher (14–30%). In these latter groups, comorbid conditions can also delay surgery or make it impossible. This can lead to complications, such as systematic sepsis and gall bladder (GB) perforation. Percutaneous cholecystostomy (PC), which was initially described by Radder in 1980, can be a safer alternative in the high-risk patients. It can also be used to access the GB for other interventions such as cholecystolithotomy and stent placement.

Diagnostic Evaluation

Clinical

- Good physical and abdominal evaluation to check for signs of acute cholecystitis and local or general peritonism.
- Full explanation of the procedure to the patient and/or family as appropriate (if patient is critically ill), including possibility of relatively long-term catheter drainage.
- Adequate antibiotic coverage.

M.S. Gulati
Department of Radiology, Queen Elizabeth Hospital & Guy's and St. Thomas' Hospitals, London, UK

D.A. Gervais and T. Sabharwal (eds.),
Interventional Radiology Procedures in Biopsy and Drainage,
DOI: 10.1007/978-1-84800-899-1_19, © Springer-Verlag London Limited 2011

Laboratory

- Full blood count, liver function tests, inflammatory laboratory parameters, and coagulation profile. Coagulation abnormalities to be corrected with platelet transfusion and/or fresh frozen plasma.

Imaging

- Ultrasonographic evaluation:
  - Presence of stones (calculus cholecystitis)
  - Ultrasonographic Murphy's sign
  - Gall bladder wall thickening
  - Pericholecystic collection/abscess
  - Debris in lumen
  - Choledocholithiasis and bile duct dilatation
  - To plan approach for cholecystostomy
- CT or MR (MRCP) if required to clarify further features

Indications

- To drain infected bile in critically ill patients who are poor candidates for surgical management (cholecystectomy). This could also be definitive for some patients in whom long-term drainage can be considered.
- As a temporizing and stabilizing measure acting as a bridge to eventual definitive cholecystectomy.
- Patients with unexplained sepsis, when all other causes have been excluded and ultrasound findings (described as above) are suggestive of acute cholecystitis. Initial puncture with a thin needle can be used to confirm this and then drainage can be done if needed.
- If there is no intrahepatic biliary dilatation and transhepatic access is difficult or not possible, cholecystostomy can be used to assess the common bile duct and to place stents across ductal obstruction.
- Access for cholecystolithotomy and percutaneous stone dissolution.

Contraindications

Absolute Contraindications

There are usually no absolute contraindications as the procedure is usually done for high-risk patients who cannot be operated immediately.
- Chialiditi's situation with interposed bowel precluding any access.
- Severe bleeding diathesis.

Relative Contraindications

- A GB completely packed with stones preventing safe formation of a self-retaining loop and locking
- GB cancer with risk of seeding of track.
- Decompressed GB due to perforation.

Relevant Anatomy and Approach

- GB is attached to the liver at the "bare area" of the liver, which is extraperitoneal. Thus, transhepatic approach has theoretical advantage of reducing risk of bile leakage.
- If this involves intercostal puncture, care should be taken to introduce the needle/catheter just above the rib to avoid damaging the intercostal vessels or nerve. Interposed bowel loops should be looked for and carefully avoided.
- Direct transperitoneal approach may occasionally be needed if transhepatic approach is not possible, for example, presence of adjacent tumor, interposed bowel.

Advantages of Transhepatic Approach

1. Extraperitoneal approach leads to less chance of bile leakage.
2. Transhepatic tract is more secure and stable as GB is less mobile here and it is easier to target even small gall bladders through this approach.
3. Transhepatic tract matures faster.

Equipment

Imaging Guidance

- Ideally ultrasound guidance should be used. A 5–8 MHz transducer is selected, which could be curved array, but preferably be a sector probe, especially if intercostal approach is used.
- Ideally C-arm image intensifier should be available unless it is a bedside procedure in a critically ill patient.
- Occasionally CT guidance maybe required if safe access under ultrasound guidance is not feasible.

Medication

- Sedation and analgesia using Fentanyl and Midazolam combination intravenously.
- Local anesthetic – 1% Lidocaine infiltrated throughout the tract – intradermal, abdominal wall, capsule of the liver, and the GB wall

- Infection control by adequate broad-spectrum antibiotics based on local guidelines.
- Contrast material to outline the GB and to confirm the intraluminal position and to check for patency of the cystic duct.

Hardware Requirements

- Neff percutaneous access micropuncture set or a 22-G Chiba needle along with a Jefferey wire guide exchange set.
- 18G puncture needle
- 0.018 in. wire (comes with triaxial Neff set)
- 0.035 in. 145 cm Rosen wire or short 0.035 in. 75 cm Amplatz super-stiff wire
- Pigtail drainage catheter, preferably with a suture-activated locking mechanism
- Drainage bag
- Adhesive disc for catheter fixation or 2–0 nylon suture

Procedure

- As mentioned previously, this procedure is ideally done under ultrasound guidance in a fluoroscopy suite with a C-arm to facilitate confirmation of GB access by contrast injection and to look for patency of cystic duct. However, in a critically ill patient, only ultrasound guidance maybe used, when the procedure has to be done at the bedside.
- Depending on best visualization (as elaborated earlier) a transhepatic (preferable) or a transperitoneal approach is chosen. The approach could be subcostal or intercostal and is usually a balance of the shortest and the safest route. This is marked on the skin.
- The chosen skin entry site is thoroughly cleaned and draped. The ultrasound probe is covered in a sterile sleeve and sterile coupling gel is used over it.
- If required, conscious sedation is used and 1% Lidocaine is injected under ultrasound guidance at the marked site, up to the GB wall and at the level of the capsule of liver (if transhepatic approach).
- A small incision is made in the skin and adequate subcutaneous incision widening is undertaken with a curved dissection forceps.
- Further introduction of the catheter is done using one of the two standard techniques:
  (a) The Seldinger technique
  (b) The Trocar technique.

The Seldinger Technique

This is the preferred technique and is well suited for relatively small GBs and when the procedure is likely to be technically difficult.
- Dependent on the level of confidence and expected ease of procedure, a micropuncture set or 18G puncture needles is used for initial access. Bile aspiration will confirm position in GB lumen.

- A 0.035 in. guide wire is introduced through 18G puncture needle (or through sheath of the micropuncture set, which would have initially required the use of a 22G needle and 0.018 in. wire). Care is taken not to coil too much wire in the lumen, especially if stiff wire is being used, as this can lead to perforation and bile leakage or even avulsion of cystic duct. The wire should be constantly visualized on ultrasound (bedside) or on fluoroscopy (aided by initial contrast injection into the lumen of the gall bladder during introduction.
- After dilatation of the tract with sequential dilators, an 8F or 10F suture-activated self-retaining locking catheter is introduced (Fig. 1a and b).
- If an intraperitoneal approach is used, the cope catheter is initially used, which has an anchoring device to draw the GB wall up against the peritoneal surface, thus reducing the risk of bile leakage during subsequent catheter exchange or manipulation during cholecystolithotomy.

Trocar Technique

This technique is useful with an easily visualized large GB and especially with a transhepatic approach. This method provides a single step access to the GB and no wire exchanges are needed. Therefore, if technically feasible, this method should be used in bedside situations. If this technique is used for transperitoneal access of GB, anchoring device must be used.

- A triple assembly of catheter, trocar (stiffening cannula) and an innermost stylet needle (that projects through the end hole of the catheter that has been straightened out with a trocar) is used.

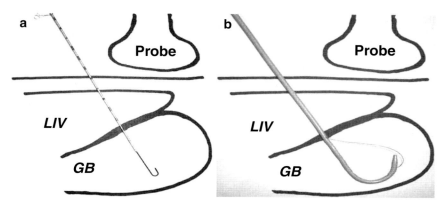

Fig. 1 (**a**) The figure shows the preferred approach to the GB while performing a transhepatic access. The needle has been inserted into the GB under ultrasound guidance and a guide wire has been introduced through it into the lumen. (**b**) After dilatation of the tract with serial dilators, a suture-activated locking pigtail catheter has been introduced into the lumen of the GB and the guide wire has been removed

- The entire system is introduced into the GB lumen under ultrasound guidance through a small incision in the skin.
- The inner stylet is removed and if in the lumen, bile can be readily aspirated from the hub of trocar (over which the catheter is still mounted).
- The drainage catheter can then simply be advanced into the lumen of the GB over the trocar, thus forming the self-retaining loop, which can be locked in place by suture activation.

With either technique, minimal (4–7 mL) amount of contrast is injected to confirm position in the GB. Larger amounts of contrast can lead to bilo-venous reflux (due to the highly inflamed mucosa) causing septicemia and bacteremia and also increase the risk of GB perforation. The catheter is fixed to the skin with a 2–0 suture or by means of an adhesive disc. Maximum possible bile should be aspirated and sent for culture and microscopic analysis. A bag is attached to the catheter for dependent drainage.

Post-procedure Care

- Gravity drainage is allowed and no flushing should be done unless there is suspicion of displacement or blockage of catheter and this should be checked under fluoroscopy and with contrast injection.
- Normally, a contrast study should be done only after 48 h to check for patency of cystic duct, to avoid bilo-venous reflux.
- The tract is allowed to mature for 3–8 weeks depending on transhepatic and transperitoneal approach.
- If tube removal is considered it should be capped for at least 48 h on a trial basis to see if the symptoms of cholecystitis will recur, and if the cystic duct remains patent. The tube should not be removed for 6 weeks until a mature track forms between the skin and the gallbladder. The tube can be removed over a 0.035 in. guide wire. Some interventional radiologists prefer to regularly perform tract evaluation by injecting contrast using a Y-connector as the catheter is being removed over the guide wire. This enables replacement of the catheter in the event of a significant bile leak from an immature tract.

Complications

- Bile leakage and GB perforation
- Avulsion of cystic duct
- Vaso-vagal reactions
- Injury/avulsion of cystic artery with life-threatening hemorrhage
- Haemobilia (usually self-limiting), or pseudoaneurysm, which may require endovascular management
- Pneumothorax, bilothorax

- Bowel injury resulting from interposed loops getting injured
- Bacteraemia, sepsis
- Tube displacement

Outcomes

It is difficult to assess results of percutaneous cholecystostomy due to a great degree of variation of patient population, demographics, and differences in type and extent of underlying illnesses. Therefore, morbidity or mortality is difficult to attribute to a particular factor. In general, most studies focus on critically ill and elderly patients.

Good technical success (more than 90%) is reported by most of the authors. Clinical success is more dependent on comorbid conditions and to what extent the presumed acute cholecystitis is contributing to the patient's condition. In general, patients with symptoms related to the right upper quadrant and those having gallstones are the ones likely to improve (and rapidly) with this procedure. Therefore, the clinical success varies from 60% to 90% with this procedure.

Percutaneous Cholecystolithotomy

- Percutaneous Cholecystolithotomy (PCCL) is a logical extension of the initial step of percutaneous cholecystectomy, particularly in patients who are elderly and/or have significant operative risks from underlying comorbid conditions.
- Many of these patients may have additional calculi, which may have slipped into the intrahepatic and extrahepatic ducts. The latter calculi may or may not be accessible for endoscopic retrograde cholangiopancreatography techniques, but could be amenable to extraction by percutaneous techniques.

Important Considerations

- Any coagulopathy should be corrected as large transhepatic tracts can bleed significantly.
- Patients should be consented and prepped in the same manner as described previously and good broad-spectrum antibiotic coverage should be provided.
- For chronic cholecystitis condition the PCCL and tract dilatation is done 24–48 h after initial drain placement.
- Whenever PCCL is a consideration (or could be considered at a later stage), the initial needle puncture should ideally be in the fundus, opposite, and as far away from the neck as possible to facilitate easy extraction with instrumentation.

Hardware Requirements

This presumes that the patient has a cholecystostomy catheter in place and the materials required for cholecystostomy have been discussed previously in the chapter. Additional requirements are as follows:

- Coaxial Teflon dilators (Cook Inc) with the largest dilators of 18 Fr size.
- A flexible choledochoscope with an outer diameter of 15F and a working channel that admits various instruments with shaft diameters up to 5F.
- Baskets and graspers compatible with the choledochoscope.
- For larger stones intracorporeal electrohydraulic lithotripsy (EHL) electrode and shock-wave generator is used.
- Some people prefer the use of smaller 11 Fr choledochoscope, which requires small access but has a smaller working channel that may not allow passage of some instruments. This scope admits laser lithotripter device to fragment the stones, which is relatively more expensive.
- Other people may use ultrasound lithotripsy, which requires a much larger access.

Procedure

- After the initial drain is removed over a guide wire, a sheath is introduced to facilitate placement of an additional safety guide wire to secure a "fall-back" access. The first guide wire is used to dilate the track to 18 Fr size using coaxial Teflon dilators and the outer 18F sheath is then secured.
- Using baskets through the sheath small stones can be removed and somewhat larger ones can be fragmented. Those that are difficult to fragment can be dealt with by EHL probe under direct vision using the choledochoscope.
- It is important to avoid injury to the biliary endothelial lining as this can lead to bile leak or bleeding (with consequent poor visualization of the field).
- After the stones are believed to have been removed, a final inspection of the lumen should be done to exclude any residual calculi. A fluoroscopic contrast study is very useful at this stage to establish patency of the cystic duct and to look for further calculi in cystic or the rest of the bile ducts.
- At the end of the procedure, a large pigtail catheter (up to 16Fr) is left in the lumen of the GB with a locking loop, to enable good drainage of bile and debris into a gravity bag and to tamponade the tract and prevent bleeding that may otherwise occur.

Results

- The success rate for complete removal has been variously reported from 70% to 100% in different series. It is critical to carefully examine the GB lumen by using both the choledochoscopic direct inspection and by fluoroscopic contrast injection methods to avoid incomplete clearance.

- The overall stone recurrence rate was 31% at a mean follow-up of 26 months in one series. However, nearly half of these patients remained asymptomatic.
- In a large series of 439 cases with a 10-year follow-up, the overall recurrence was seen in 41.4% patients and again nearly half of these remained asymptomatic. Twenty-three percent of patients with recurrent calculi had to be retreated with cholecystectomy. Therefore, PCCL should be done in carefully selected patients.

Complications

These are similar to percutaneous cholecystectomy and have been described earlier.

Key Points

> Patients who have acute cholecystitis, with or without gallstones, and have underlying significant comorbid conditions, can significantly benefit from cholecystostomy. This is relatively minimally invasive and safe and can be definitive in many situations, in particular, acalculous cholecystitis.
> Access to GB should preferably be transhepatic and under ultrasound guidance with fluoroscopy assistance and using Seldinger technique, although in bedside situations this can be modified as suggested based on technical considerations.
> Percutaneous cholecystostomy provides opportunities in select situations for cholecystolithotomy and other more complex biliary ductal procedures, especially when risks from surgery in such situations are particularly high.

Suggested Reading

1. Akham O, Akinci D, Ozmen MN. Percutaneous cholecystostomy. *Eur J radiol*. 2002;43:229-236.
2. Winbladh A, Gullstrand P, Svanvik J, Sandström P. Symptomatic review of cholecystostomy as a treatment option in acute cholecystitis. *HPB (Oxford)*. 2009;11:183-193.
3. Leveau P, Andersson E, Carlgren I, Willner J, Andersson R. Percutaneous cholecystostomy: a bridge to surgery or definite management of acute cholecystitis in high-risk patients? *Scand J Gastroenterol*. 2008;43:593-596.
4. Cheslyn-Curtis S, Gillams AR, Russell RC, et al. Selection, management, and early outcome of 113 patients with symptomatic gallstones treated by percutaneous cholecystolithotomy. *Gut*. 1992;33:1253-1259.
5. Malone DE. Interventional alternatives to cholecystectomy. *Radiol Clin North Am*. 1990;28:1145-1156.
6. Zou YP, Du JD, Li WM, et al. Gallstone recurrence after successful percutaneous cholecysto-lithotomy: a 10 year follow-up of 439 cases. *Hepatobiliary Pancreat Dis Int*. 2007;6:199-203.

Percutaneous Nephrostomy and Antegrade Ureteric Stenting

Sundeep Punamiya

Percutaneous Nephrostomy

Clinical Features

Symptoms of upper urinary tract obstruction include flank or abdominal pain, nausea, vomiting, and fever (if urinary tract infection); seldom aysmptomatic (incidentally diagnosed on imaging or during evaluation of urinary tract infection).

If obstruction involves a solitary functioning kidney or both kidneys simultaneously, symptoms of acute renal failure (oliguria/anuria, nausea, vomiting, pedal edema, and altered sensorium) may be noted. May also be complicated by symptoms related to electrolyte imbalance and acidosis.

Diagnostic Evaluation

- Clinical
  - History to establish cause of obstruction
  - Evaluate complications such as sepsis, renal failure, electrolyte imbalance, and acidosis
  - Clinical examination: Evaluate vital parameters, renal angle tenderness, surgical scars, and body habitus predicting difficult access/positioning
- Laboratory
  Bleeding and exacerbation of urinary infection are the most feared complications of PCN
  - FBC and coagulation profile
  - Urinalysis (look for active UTI)
  - Renal profile

S. Punamiya
Diagnostic Radiology Department, Tan Tock Seng Hospital, Singapore

D.A. Gervais and T. Sabharwal (eds.),
Interventional Radiology Procedures in Biopsy and Drainage,
DOI: 10.1007/978-1-84800-899-1_20, © Springer-Verlag London Limited 2011

- Imaging
  - Intravenous urogram, US, and/or CT are always done to confirm indication for PCN, and evaluate degree of dilatation of pelvicalyceal system, position of kidney, and selection of optimal approach.

Indications

1. Urinary tract obstruction
   (a) Malignancy (commonly cervical, prostatic, metastatic pelvic adenopathy, urothelial)
   (b) Stone
   (c) Ureteric or anastomotic stricture
   (d) Pyonephrosis
   (e) Assessment of functional recovery of obstructed kidney
2. Urinary diversion
   (a) Ureteral injury
   (b) Vesical fistula
   (c) Hemorrhagic cystitis
3. Access for subsequent interventional or endoscopic procedures
   (a) Removal of renal or ureteral calculi
   (b) Antegrade ureteral stenting
   (c) Dilatation of ureteral or anastomotic stricture
   (d) Endopyelotomy
   (e) Deliver medications (fungal ball, urothelial tumors, stone dissolution)
   (f) Ureteral occlusion for refractory leak
   (g) Biopsy of urothelial lesion
   (h) Foreign body retrieval

Relative Contraindications

1. Uncontrolled coagulopathy
   (a) INR > 1.3
   (b) aPTT > 1.5 times normal
   (c) Platelet count < $50–100 \times 10^9$/L
2. Anticoagulant therapy (aspirin, heparin, warfarin)
3. Uncontrolled hypertension
4. Terminal illness, imminent death

Patient Preparation

1. Antibiotic prophylaxis in high-risk cases
2. Correction of hyperkalemia and/or metabolic acidosis, if any

Relevant Anatomy

Normal Anatomy

1. Kidneys are rotated, with coronal plane of kidney 30–50° to the coronal plane of the body. Also, upper pole of the kidney lies more medial than the lower pole.
2. Kidney has four coverings, of which the Gerota's fascia and true capsule are two areas of resistance during needle puncture. Renal capsule is richly innervated and if unanesthetized can be a cause of severe pain.
3. The pelvicalceal system typically consists of 14 calyces (range 4–28). The upper and lower calyces are usually compound and oriented in a polar direction. The remaining calyces are arranged in two distinct rows: anterior and posterior. Anterior calyces form an angle of 70° with the frontal plane of the kidney and the posterior calyces form an angle of 20°. This pattern, when combined with the normal rotation of the kidneys, projects the anterior calyces side-on (cup-shaped) while the posterior calyces are seen end-on (circular).
4. The renal artery divides into an anterior and posterior division, which creates an avascular zone between them (Brodel's line of incision). This zone is 1–2 cm posterior to the lateral margin of the kidney. Needle track through this zone will encounter least bleeding (Figs.1 and 2).

Aberrant Anatomy

1. Malrotated and horseshoe kidneys would orient the posterior calyx more medially, necessitating a puncture through the paraspinal muscles.

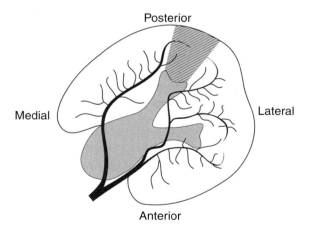

Fig. 1 Cross-section of the kidney showing the relationship between the arteries and pelvicalyceal system. The avascular zone of Brodel lies between the anterior and posterior segments of the kidney. Needle traversal through this zone to access the posterior calyx is least likely to cause bleeding

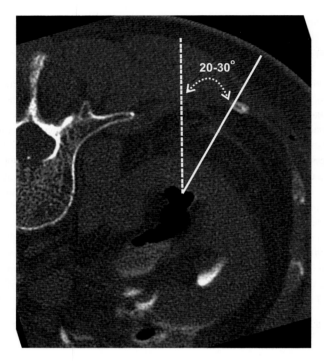

Fig. 2 Needle trajectory (*solid line*) is directed toward the posterior calyx, about 20–30% from the sagittal plane of patient (*interrupted line*), to ensure passage through the avascular zone of Brodel

Transplant Anatomy

1. Transplant kidney is placed in the extra peritoneal space in the right iliac fossa, with the pelvis oriented medially and calyces laterally.

Equipment

1. Needles: 21G Chiba needle, 18G initial puncture needle, fine-needle coaxial set (Accustick, Neff)
2. Guide wires: "0.018" Cope mandril wire, "0.035" hydrophilic wire, "0.035" stiff Amplatz wire
3. Catheters: 8F or 10F pigtail drainage catheters, 30–45 cm long, preferably with self-retaining mechanism

Procedure

Imaging Guidance

1. Can be done using fluroscopy, US, or CT alone or in combination. Best success rates and safety profiles are achieved when PCN is performed using a combination of US and fluroscopy. CT guidance may be preferred in malrotated kidneys, horseshoe kidneys, retrorenal colon, marked kyphoscoliosis, and body habitus that prevents optimal positioning of patient.
2. In case of urinary leak/fistula, the pelvicalyceal system is not dilated, making calyceal puncture very difficult with US/CT. In this situation, intravenous contrast can be injected to opacify the system prior to puncture using fluoroscopic guidance.

Positioning the Patient

1. Optimally prone position. If not possible, a prone-oblique position may be attempted, with the ipsilateral side up.
2. For transplant kidneys PCN is attempted with patient in the supine position.

Planning an Access Route

1. Important to avoid trauma or access through major renal vessels, pleura, colon, and spleen.
2. The posterior calyx needs to be punctured close to its tip, preferably at its junction with infundibulum. A postero-lateral approach is used, with the needle directed medially about 20–30° to the patient's sagittal plane (Figs. 1and 2).
3. Choice of calyx depends on the indication and subsequent planned therapy.
4. If PCN is being performed for the sole purpose of external drainage, any posterior calyx can be selected for puncture. However, if subsequent stenting is planned or is a distinct possibility, a mid or upper calyx would be preferred. If stone removal is planned through the PCN tract, choice of calyx will depend on location of stone.
5. In transplant kidneys, the kidney is accessed from an anterior approach. The lateral calyx is chosen for puncture, to avoid peritoneal transgression and its associated problems such as cecal and vacular injury.

Performing the Procedure

Technique

1. Double-stick method
   First step: A 22G Chiba needle is advanced directly into the renal pelvis from a posterior approach through renal angle, using US or fluroscopy. Correct entry into pelvi-

calyceal system is confirmed with aspiration of urine and injection of contrast. Take care that the volume of urine aspirated is more than the volume of contrast injected, to avoid over distension and potential bacteremia.

Second step: An appropriate posterior calyx is selected for puncture. This may need an additional injection of air/CO_2 through the Chiba needle, as the posterior calyx is non-dependent and may not be seen on injection of iodinated contrast. Micropuncture set or an 18G initial puncture needle is then used to access the posterior calyx, following which a guidewire is inserted and coiled in the renal pelvis, then tract dilatation is done with dilators, and an 8–10 F pigtail drainage catheter is inserted.

2. Single-stick method

With this method, there is no need to obtain an antegrade pyelogram prior to calyceal puncture. Here, the posterior calyx is selected on US or CT, and punctured with real-time imaging guidance, with either the micropuncture set or the 18G initial puncture needle. The remaining procedure is conducted as mentioned in the second step of a double-stick technique, preferably using fluoroscopy as guidance.

End-point

Procedural end-point is when the catheter is adequately coiled in the renal pelvis, and confirmed with a small amount of contrast injection.

Immediate Post-Procedure Care

1. Bed rest 4 h.
2. Monitor vital parameters q30 min for 2 h, then q1 h for 4 h.
3. Monitor fluid input and output charts.
4. Monitor PCN output. If no output, inspect tubing and connections for blockage by blood clots/thick pus/debris, and kinks; may need gentle irrigation with 5–10 mL saline.
5. Monitor hematuria. Hematuria expected upto 48 h, slowly clearing over this period. If hematuria gross or persists beyond 48 h, check catheter position, hematocrit, coagulation parameters. Consider angiogram and embolization if arterial bleeding suspected (severe or intermittent hematuria).
6. Continue antibiotics if urosepsis.
7. Analgesics PRN.

Follow-Up and Post-Procedure Medications

1. PCN drainage to be continued till obstruction is relieved with surgery, stenting, etc.
2. If on long-term drainage, to provide instructions on catheter care:
    (a) Daily dressing over catheter entry site
    (b) Can bathe with care to keep catheter entry site dry. No tub or pool baths

(c) Regular emptying of urine from the drainage bag
(d) Contact radiology service if:
    (i) Reduced drainage from PCN.
    (ii) Fever, flank pain, or pericatheteral leak.
    (iii) PCN catheter appears to have pulled out.
(e) Change of PCN catheter q3 months.

Results

1. Technical success rate for dilated system >95%.
2. Technical success rate for non-dilated system >80%.
3. Technical success date for complex or staghorn stones >85%.
4. Mortality rate 0.04%.
5. Overall complication rate approximately 10%.
6. Major complications requiring transfer to ICU, emergency salvage procedure (surgery/embolization), or delayed discharge from hospital <5%.

Alternative Therapies

Retrograde ureteral stenting

Complications

1. Sepsis seen in 1–3% of cases; the incidence increases to 7–9% in patients with pre-existing pyonephrosis.
2. Hemorrhage (hematuria, retroperitoneal hematoma, subcasular hematoma) noted in 1–4%. However, the need for transcatheter embolization or surgery to control bleeding is required in <1%.
3. Pleural complications (pneumothorax, empyema, hydrothorax, hemothorax) is seen in 0.1–0.2% cases usually when a supracostal puncture is used.
4. Injury to adjacent organs (spleen, liver, colon) is rare.

How to Avoid

1. Correct coagulopathy.
2. Administer prophylactic antibiotics.
3. Review images of prior radiological investigations for anatomic variations, retrorenal colon.
4. Continuous monitoring of needle passage with fluoroscopy, US, or CT fluoroscopy.
5. Puncture below 11th rib to avoid transgressing pleura.

6. Needle approach to the tip of posterior calyx should be postero-lateral, with a 20–30° angle from vertical, to avoid major blood vessel.
7. Do not overdistend system with contrast if system is infected.
8. Avoid prolonged or complicated procedure if system is infected.
9. Use self-retaining catheters to prevent accidental extrusion.

Antegrade Ureteric Stenting

Indications

Antegrade stenting is considered when retrograde stenting has failed, or stenting is now considered in a patient with an indwelling PCN. Indications for stenting include:
1. Relief of ureteric obstruction from any cause (stone, stricture, external compression, etc.)
2. Ureteric fistula
3. Ureteric trauma
4. Prior to endocorporeal shock wave lithotropsy (solitary kidney or large stone >15 mm)
5. Post ureteroscopy
6. Post ureteric reconstruction

Contraindications

1. Untreated bladder outlet obstruction
2. Vesical fistula
3. Urinary incontinence
4. Small, irritable bladder
5. Bladder tumors
6. Active urinary tract infection
7. Significant bleeding following PCN

Patient Preparation

1. Antegrade stenting is usually done about 2–7 days after insertion of PCN. This has several advantages:
   (a) It is easier to traverse the obstruction as the edema at obstruction site subsides and the ureteric dilatation and tortuousity is reduced.
   (b) PCN tract maturation would make manipulation for stent insertion less traumatic.
   (c) Urine is clear of infection and/or hematuria, resulting in longer stent function.
2. There are some centers that proceed to one stage ureteric stenting with good results and strict adherence to good technique is vital for this practice.
3. Antibiotic prophylaxis: cefazolin 1 g single-dose before procedure.
4. If patients had urinary tract infection, culture-specific antibiotics are administered at least 5 days prior to allow urine to be sterile.

Equipment

1. Guidewires: 0.035′ hydrophilic wire, 0.035″ Teflon wire, 0.035″ Amplatz wire
2. Sheath: 1 F larger than the stent being used, and at least 25 cm long
3. Catheter: 4–5 F Kumpe access catheter, Berenstein or BMC catheter to provide directional control of the guidewire
4. Ureteral stent: 6 F or 7 F

Pre-procedure Medication

1. Antibiotics
2. Analgesia/sedation: As for PCN

Procedure

Imaging Guidance

1. Always done under fluoroscopy.

Positioning the Patient

1. Optimally prone position. If not possible, a prone-oblique position may be attempted, with the ipsilateral side up.
2. For transplant kidneys stenting is attempted with patient in the supine position.

Technique

1. Local anesthetic is infiltrated around entry site of the PCN catheter.
2. Nephrostogram is obtained by injecting contrast through the indwelling PCN catheter, and the site of obstruction is determined.
3. PCN catheter is removed over a guidewire. Remember to release the anchoring suture if the PCN catheter has a Cope-loop.
4. The catheter is exchanged for a sheath that is advanced as distally as possible. The sheath will reduce the trauma of manipulation associated with crossing the ureteric obstruction. In addition, it provides support for passage of catheter/stent across the angulation at the renal pelvis, especially when the approach is from an inferior calyx.
5. A 4–5 F curved catheter is advanced through the sheath to the level of obstruction.
6. A hydrophilic wire is used to cross the obstruction, and advanced into the bladder. The catheter is advanced over it into the bladder. Entry into the bladder is confirmed with contrast injection.
7. A Teflon or Amplatz wire is inserted and catheter removed.

8. The ureteric stent is then advanced over the wire and deployed in the following manner:
   (a) When the distal end of the stent is within the bladder, the wire is partially with-
       drawn to release the pre-formed J loop of the stent in the bladder.
   (b) The wire is then withdrawn further up to the renal pelvis, after which the stent
       pusher is used to advance the stent into the pelvis and form the proximal loop.
       Remember to retract the sheath into the calyx before deploying the stent.
9. The wire is disengaged from the stent, and re-advanced into the pelvis, and a catheter
   is inserted for temporary decompression.
10. This temporary catheter is removed after an overnight trial of clamping. Catheter can
    be removed if there is no pericatheteral leak, fever, or flank pain. Stent function may
    be confirmed by a nephrostogram prior to removal of catheter.

Choosing the Stent

1. Length of stent: It is important to choose an appropriate stent length to prevent irritative
   voiding symptoms. Stents are available in a wide range of fixed lengths, ranging
   between 20 and 28 cm. Multi-length stents are also available. Length of stent required
   is estimated by any of the following methods:
   (a) *Height of patient*:

<5′10″	22 cm
5′10″–6′4″	24 cm
>6′4″	26 cm

   (b) *Wire measure*: Once catheter–wire combination has crossed the ureter into the blad-
       der, the wire is withdrawn under fluoroscopy, marking it externally at two points:
       (i) when the wire tip is at the ureterovesical junction and (ii) when the wire tip is in
       the renal pelvis. The marking can be done by either bending the wire at these two
       points or with artery forceps clamped on the wire at these two points. The length of
       wire between these two points, when measured with a ruler, determines the stent
       length.
   (c) Calibrated wire or catheter.
2. Anchoring system
   (a) Double J stent (J loop on either end): Pigtail loop on either end reduces migration
       rate and is the commonest type of stent used. The loop in the bladder can produce
       significant trigonal irritation and discomfort.
   (b) Tail stent (J loop on upper end and straight at lower end): The short intravesical
       segment of this stent reduces the irritative symptoms of the stent coil in the bladder
       (Polaris, Boston Scientific).
3. Material of stent.
   (a) Silicone: Lowest encrustation rate, but high co-efficient of friction, soft and diffi-
       cult to insert through tight strictures (Fluoro-4, Bard).
   (b) Polyurethane: Stiffer and easier to introduce, but high rate of encrustation.

(c) Co-polymers: Newest material, lower rate of encrustation, easy to introduce. Includes material like Percuflex (Boston Scientific), C-flex (Cook).

(d) Metal stents: Reduces the stent dysfunction due to external compression by bulky tumors (Resonance, Cook).

End-Point

Procedural end-point is when the stent is appropriately positioned, with distal end coiled in the bladder, and proximal end coiled in the renal pelvis. Stent function is assessed with contrast injection through the temporary catheter.

Immediate Post-Procedure Care

1. Bed rest 4 h.
2. Monitor vital parameters q1 h for 4 h.
3. Monitor fluid input and output charts.
4. Monitor PCN output.
5. Monitor hematuria. Mild hematuria is expected upto 48 h.
6. Analgesics prn.
7. Clamp the temporary drain overnight. Monitor for signs of stent dysfunction, namely, pericatheter leak, flank pain and/or fever. The drain would need to be released if any of these signs are evident during this trial of clamping. A check nephrostogram would be needed to assess stent function next day.

Follow-Up and Post-Procedure Medication

1. Stents are not permanent implants and ideally need to be removed within 6 weeks.
2. If long-term stent is planned, retrograde change of DJ stent q12 weeks.
3. Oral ciprofloxacin may be given for 3 days every 2 weeks to reduce bacterial colonization of stent.
4. Abdominal X-ray to check position of stent if irritative voiding symptoms persist or suspicion of stent dysfunction.

Results

Success rate of antegrade stent insertion is 88–96%. Success is lowest for benign, occlusive strictures (e.g., post-radiation, tubercular, and post-operative strictures).

Alternative Therapies

1. Nephroureterostomy catheter
2. Extra-anatomic stents
3. Long-term PCN

Complications

Early Complications

1. Lower abdominal pain
2. Irritative voiding symptoms (urinary frequency, dysuria, and nocturia)
3. Hematuria, usually microscopic
4. Urinary infection
5. Acute stent blockage (flank pain, fever, leak from PCN site)

Late Complications

1. Stent migration
2. Stent encrustation and blockage
3. Ureteral erosion or fistulization
4. Stent fragmentation
5. Forgotten stent

How to Avoid

1. Approach from a mid-polar calyx rather than an inferior polar calyx.
2. Use stent of correct length, avoid a long intravesical segment.
3. Softer stents are better tolerated.
4. Stage the stent placement at least 2–7 days after PCN, and to be attempted only after urine is clear.
5. Ensure stent is removed or exchanged within 12 weeks before marked encrustation occurs.

Key Points

> Successful and uncomplicated PCN and ureteric stenting requires evaluation of the renal anatomy with imaging prior to renal puncture.
> Using a combination of US and fluoroscopy will provide the best results.
> Puncture needle should be directed toward the posterior calyx and not the pelvis.
> Trajectory through the kidney should be along the avascular zone of Brodel to avoid major bleeding.

Suggested Reading

1. Dyer RB, Regan JD, Kavanagh PV, Khatod EG, Chen MY, Zagoria RJ. Percutaneous nephrostomy with extensions of the technique: step by step. *Radiographics*. 2002;22:503-525.
2. Millward SF. Percutaneous nephrostomy: a practical approach. *J Vasc Interv Radiol*. 2000;11:955-964.
3. Hausegger KA, Portugaller HR. Percutaneous nephrostomy and antegrade ureteral stenting: technique-indications-complications. *Eur Radiol*. 2006;16:2016-2030.
4. Zagoria RJ, Dyer RB. Do's and don't's of percutaneous nephrostomy. *Acad Radiol*. 1999;6: 370-377.
5. Kaye KW. Renal anatomy: Endourological considerations. In: Clayman RV, Castaneda-Zuniga WR, eds. *Techniques in Endourology: A Guide to the Percutaneous Removal of Renal and Ureteral Calculi*. Chicago: Year Book Medical; 1984:55-71.
6. Dyer RB, Chen MY, Zagoria RJ, Regan JD, Hood CG, Kavanagh PV. Complications of ureteral stent placement. *Radiographics*. 2002;22:1005-1022.

Fluoroscopy-Guided Percutaneous Renal Access for Treatment of Stone Disease

Brian H. Eisner and Debra A. Gervais

Clinical Features

- Urinary stone disease is a common cause of morbidity and mortality with a lifetime incidence of 10%.
- Several treatment modalities are commonly used to treat renal and ureteral stones, including shock wave lithotripsy (SWL), ureteroscopy, and percutaneous nephrolithotomy (PCNL).
- PCNL is standard of care for large renal pelvis stones (≥ 2 cm), lower pole stones (≥ 1.5 cm), and branched calculi which occupy multiple renal calyces (i.e., staghorn calculi).
- Of all stone treatments, PCNL carries greatest surgical risk.

Diagnostic Evaluation

Laboratory

Basic metabolic panel, complete blood count, coagulation studies, blood bank sample.

Imaging

- Some preoperative imaging is necessary (KUB, ultrasound, or CT scan).
- CT or MRI may be useful in defining anatomy.

B.H. Eisner (✉)
Department of Urology, Massachusetts General Hospital, Harvard Medical School, Boston, MA, USA

D.A. Gervais and T. Sabharwal (eds.),
Interventional Radiology Procedures in Biopsy and Drainage,
DOI: 10.1007/978-1-84800-899-1_21, © Springer-Verlag London Limited 2011

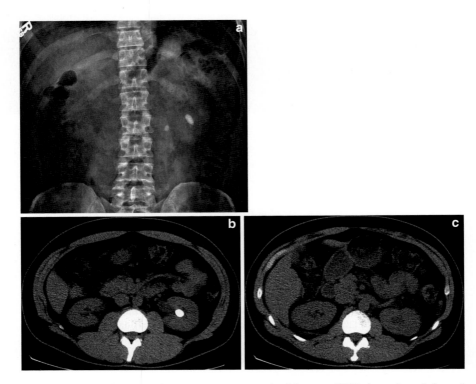

Fig. 1 Preoperative imaging prior to percutaneous nephrolithotomy. KUB shows 2 cm left renal pelvis stone and 1 cm left upper ureteral stone (**a**). Axial CT images show that there are no adjacent organs lying within the potential percutaneous tract for a lower pole puncture (**b**) or an upper pole puncture (**c**)

- — Proximity of upper pole of kidney to pleura
- — Proximity of kidney to spleen, liver, colon (Fig. 1)

Indications

- Large renal pelvis stones (≥2 cm).
- Lower pole stones (≥1.5 cm).
- Branched stones occupying several renal calyces (i.e., staghorn calculi).
- Multiple small stones so that total stone burden is large (≥2 cm).
- Stones refractory to SWL and ureteroscopy
- Patients in whom retrograde access and ureteroscopy cannot be performed (i.e., urinary diversion).

Alternative Therapies

- Shock wave lithotripsy (SWL)
- Ureteroscopy
- Laparoscopic or open stone surgery

Contraindications

- Coagulopathy/bleeding diathesis
- Anti-coagulation medications

Specific Complications

- Bleeding (sometimes requiring transfusion, embolization, or nephrectomy)
- Injury to adjacent organs (liver, spleen, colon, duodenum)
- Injury to pleura and lung (more common for upper pole access)
- Perforation of renal collecting system and urinary extravasation
- Renal infundibular stenosis or ureteral stricture
- Infections/sepsis

Anatomy

- Kidney and adjacent organs
  — Pleura – majority of supracostal access will traverse pleura; some infra-costal upper-pole punctures will traverse pleura.
  — Liver and spleen – risk of injury greatest at full or mid inspiration.
  — Colon – risk of injury greatest for retrorenal colon.
- Pelvicalyceal system
  — Upper pole calyces most commonly oriented mediolaterally.
  — Lower pole calyces most commonly oriented antero-posterior.
  — Entry into posterior-facing calyx is desired for optimal maneuverability of nephroscope and stone extraction.
- Intrarenal vasculature
  — Segmental and intralobular (infundibular) arteries run in-between calyces.
  — Safest puncture site to minimize bleeding is directly through a minor calyx (Fig. 2).

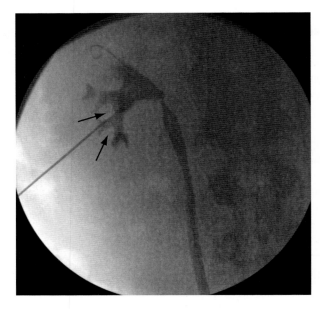

Fig. 2 Puncture directly into calyx avoids segmental and intralobar arteries. Position of arteries denoted by *arrows*

Equipment

- Retrograde placement of ureteral catheter
    — Flexible cystoscope
    — Guidewire
    — 5 F open-ended ureteral catheter
    — Radio-opaque contrast agent for injection
- Percutaneous puncture
    — Two-part entry needle for guidewire introduction
        — 18G to indtroduce 0.035 or 0.038-in. guidewire
        — 21G to introduce 0.018-in. guidewire
- Guidewires
    — Standard PTFE
    — Moveable core PTFE
    — Hydrophillic
    — Extra-stiff
- Safety-wire introduction
    — Dual-lumen catheter
    — Coaxial dilator set
- Tract dilation
    — Coaxial dilators
    — Dilation balloon

- Tamponade balloon
  — Tamponade balloon nephrostomy can be used for severe bleeding
- Medications
  — Preoperative intravenous antibiotics
  — Mannitol (theoretically can decrease bleeding)

Access Technique

- First step is always cystoscopic placement of ureteral cathether for retrograde opacification of the renal collecting system (supine or prone).
- Patient is then positioned prone (if not already done).
- Two commonly used techniques for access.
  — Bull's-eye
  — Triangulation
- Bull's-eye technique.
  — Rotate C-arm *image* 90° from standard upright position
    — Clockw*ise rotation for right access*
    — *Counter*clockwise rotation for left access
  — Rotate C-arm 30° toward surgeon
    — Target posterior calyx with "bulls-eye configuration"
    — Make stab incision in skin
    — 18G needle used to enter collecting system with bulls-eye configuration maintained
    — To assess depth of puncture, rotate C-arm back to upright position
- Triangulation technique.
  — Upright (antero-posterior) projection of C-arm used to make left-right alignments and adjustments.
  — Oblique projection of C-arm used to make adjustments of depth.
  — After alignment, needle is advanced with C-arm in oblique orientation.
- Confirmation of entry into collecting system.
  — Urine drips or is aspirated from needle
  — Inject needle with dilute contrast
  — Able to feel stone with tip of needle
  — Advance guidewire through needle into collecting system
- Initial guidewire placement.
  — PTFE guidewire is often adequate; moveable core allows operator to "coil" large amount of wire in renal pelvis if desired.
  — Hydrophilic wires useful if stone is difficult to bypass or occupies large portion of collecting system.
  — If access down the ureter is desired, 5 F angiographic catheter is used.
- Safety-wire placement.
  — 8/10 F coaxial dilator or dual-lumen cathether can be used for placement of safety wire

- Tract dilation.
  - Dilate percutaneous tract up to 24–30 F with coaxial fascial dilators or balloon dilators
    - Balloon pressures range from 15 to 30 atm.
  - Coaxial dilators more difficult to use in obese patients because of perinephric guidewire buckling
- After tract is dilated and sheath is in place, stone fragmentation and/or extraction may begin.

Key Points

> Percutaneous nephrolithotomy is standard treatment for large renal stones.
> Direct entry into calyx avoids intrarenal arteries.
> Posterior-oriented calyx is optimal for maneuvering of nephroscope.

Safety

> Care must be taken in patients with bleeding disorders.
> Anti-coagulation medications must be held if possible.

Suggested Reading

Initial Chapters of This book!

1. Kothary N, Soulen M, Clark T, Wein A, Shlansky-Goldberg R, Crino P, Stavropoulos W. Renal Angiomyolipoma: Long-term Results after Arterial Embolization J Vasc Interv Radiol 2005
2. Rimon U, Duvdevani, Garniek A, Golan G, Bensaid P, Ramon J, Morag B. Large renal angiomyolipomas: digital subtraction angiographic grading and presentation with bleeding. Clin Rad 2006; 520-526

Percutaneous Gastrostomy and Gastrojejunostomy

Philip J. Haslam

Clinical Features

Gastrostomy or gastrojejunostomy is usually needed in patients requiring enteral feeding for more than 2 weeks either due to impaired swallowing or oesophageal abnormality contraindicating a nasogastric tube.

Diagnostic Evaluation

Clinical

- Check for the abscence of hepatomegally, ascites, disseminated intra-abdominal malignancy.
- A history of previous gastric/ulcer surgery is important; partial gastrectomy and gastro-enterostomy can make the procedure more difficult.
- Full explanation of the procedure, feeding regime, alternatives, and its risks should be given during the consent process.
- Involvement of dieticians is essential.

Laboratory

- Full blood count, coagulation studies

P.J. Haslam
Department of Radiology, Freeman Hospital, Newcastle-Upon-Tyne, UK

D.A. Gervais and T. Sabharwal (eds.),
Interventional Radiology Procedures in Biopsy and Drainage,
DOI: 10.1007/978-1-84800-899-1_22, © Springer-Verlag London Limited 2011

Imaging

- Ultrasound to assess the medial extent of the liver can be useful if not clinically apparent.

Indications

Prolonged enteral feeding requirement usually due to:
- Oropharyngeal carcinoma
- Inoperable/unstentable oesophageal carcinoma
- Stroke
- Degenerative neurological conditions such as motor neurone disease
- Gastric decompression

Contraindictaions

Absolute

- Ascites
- Peritonitis
- Small bowel obstruction
- Disseminated intra-abdominal malignancy
- Portal hypertension with gastric varices

Relative

- Bleeding diathesis
- Previous gastric surgery
- Active gastric ulceration
- Pregnancy

Patient Preparation

- An NG tube should be placed prior to the procedure.
- 200 mL dilute barium may be given the night before to highlight the colon.
- Nil by mouth for 2 h prior to the procedure.

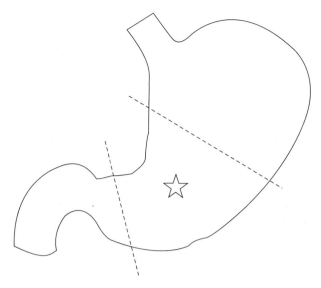

Fig. 1 The ideal location is shown by the star

Relevant Anatomy

- The ideal location for gastrostomy is in the distal body/proximal antrum of the stomach.
- Try to locate the puncture centrally thus avoiding the more peripheral vessels (Fig. 1).

Aberrant Anatomy

1. High riding stomach under the costal margin:
   Commonest in patients with motor neurone disease.
   This makes the procedure more challenging but can usually be overcome with buscopan and adequate gastric distension with air.
2. Partial gastrectomy:
   This can be overcome providing there is sufficient stomach visible to puncture.
3. Gastroenterostomy:
   This makes it more difficult to distend the stomach as it rapidly decompresses into the jejunum. Adequate distension essential.
4. Hiatus hernia:
   A large hernia with the stomach in the chest can make the procedure almost impossible.
5. Large left lobe of liver:
   This can rarely overly the stomach and clearly needs to be avoided.

6. Overlying transverse colon:
   Frequently the colon may be seen to overly the stomach on screening. It can usually be displaced inferiorly when the stomach is fully inflated and is often seen to be posterior when screening laterally.

Equipment

Gastrostomy Tube

- Button gastrostomy tube, balloon retained (Fig. 2)
- Pigtail gastrostomy with locking loop
- Balloon-retained Foley-type catheter (Fig. 3)

Gastropexy Kit (T Fasteners)

- Balt Harpoon kit (Fig. 4) or Cook Cope Anchors (Fig. 5)

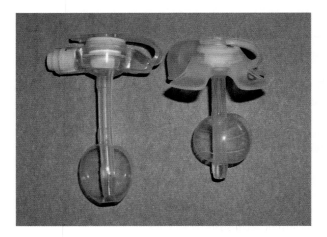

Fig. 2 Button gastrostomy tube, balloon-retained (Vygon and Corpack)

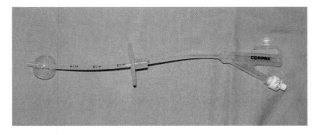

Fig. 3 Balloon-retained Foley-type catheter, (Corpack)

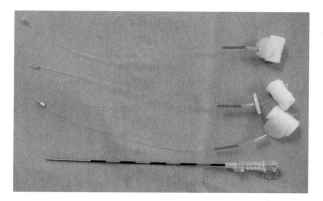

Fig. 4 Balt Harpoon kit

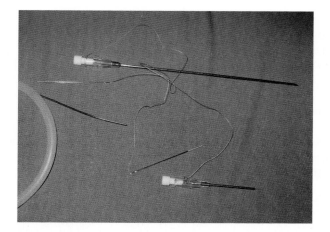

Fig. 5 Cook Cope Anchors

Stiff Guidewire

- Amplatz extra stiff or super stiff
- 8 F vascular dilator (for one step button technique)
- 6 mm angioplasty balloon

Medication

- Buscopan 20–60 mg IV. Nb contraindications
- Local anesthetic for gastropexy sites and gastrostomy puncture site
- Fentanyl IV for analgesia
- Midazolam IV for sedation

This procedure can easily be performed without sedation if necessary.

Procedure

Planning an Access Route

- Fully inflate the stomach via the NG tube post IV buscopan
- Use forceps or other metallic marker to screen position
- Aim for distal body/proximal antrum of the stomach (Fig. 6)
- Superior to the transverse colon and inferior to the costal margin (Fig. 7)

Performing the Procedure: Primary Button Gastrostomy

Gastropexy

- At least two T fasteners should be placed for a button gastrostomy.
- One could be used for a smaller balloon-retained tube or locking pigtail.
- Leave the T fasteners "snug" but not so tight they will cause post-procedure pain.

Stomach Puncture

- The area between the T fasteners is punctured with an angiographic needle or gastropexy needle.
- Insert a stiff guidewire.

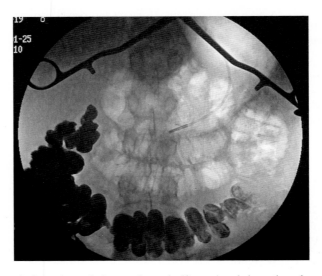

Fig. 6 The stomach shown beneath the costal margin (forceps) and above the colon

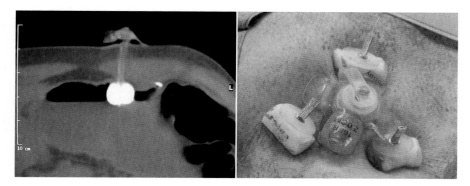

Fig. 7 The button gastrostomy in position

Measure Tract

- Insert the 6 mm angioplasty balloon and inflate in the stomach.
- Pull balloon back so in contact with gastric mucosa. Mark balloon at skin level.
- Deflate balloon and pull back into the tract so proximal balloon marker is visible.
- Measure distance between balloon marker and mark from skin level: this is the tract length.
- Select button gastrostomy of this length.

Tube Insertion

- Insert 8 F dilator into button gastrostomy tube to aid rigidity
- Firmly push gastrostomy into stomach with rotation to aid passage
- Inflate balloon (1 mL contrast 4 mL water)

Check Position

- Withdraw guidewire.
- Inject contrast using dilator while screening laterally and withdrawing.
- Contrast should flow feely into stomach and balloon should clearly be seen within gastric air. (It may still be possible to inject contrast into the stomach with the balloon in the tract.)

Performing the Procedure: Balloon- or Locking Pigtail-Retained Tubes

Easier but less desirable for the patient as not low profile and more easily blocked
- Initial procedure identical with gastropexy performed.
- Balloon-retained tubes should be inserted through a peelaway sheath due to the additional size of the balloon.
- Smaller caliber locking pigtail tubes may be inserted without a sheath.

Performing the Procedure: "Endoscopic Type" Tubes

This can be performed without gastropexy but requires the tubes to be passed per orally which is contraindicated in patients with nasopharyngeal cancer:

- The stomach is inflated then punctured percutaneously.
- A vascular 5F sheath can then be inserted over a guidewire.
- A 5F angled catheter is inserted through the sheath into the stomach.
- The esophagus is cannulated retrogradely and catheter passed out through the mouth.
- A long stiff exchange guidewire is inserted through the catheter.
- The tapered "push type" gastrostomy tube is then inserted over the wire and once visible at the skin surface can be pulled through.
- The wire is removed and the tube cut to length and fixed in place.

The advantage of this technique is the robust tube that is difficult to accidentally remove. The disadvantage is the per oral approach.

Immediate Post-Procedure Care

- Post-sedation observations and observation for hemorrhage.
- Fasting for 6 h.
- Water via gastrostomy 25 mL/h for 6 h
- Increase to 50 mL/h if no pain or other complications.
- Commence feeding regime the following day.
- T fasteners can be cut at 48 h.
- Gastrostomy tube should be rotated within stoma every 24 h.
- Balloon-retained devices should have balloon aspirated and reinflated with water every 7–10 days.

Gastrojejunostomy

Indications

- Enteral feeding in patients with:
  - Gastroesophageal reflux disease
  - Gastric outlet obstruction
- Patients needing overnight infusion feeding rather than intermittent bolus feeding

The initial procedure is the same as for standard balloon-retained gastrostomy except tract length need not be measured:

(These patients frequently have an existing gastrostomy in situ.)

- Gastropexy.
- Stomach punctured and stiff guidewire passed into jejunum.
- Tract dilated to appropriate size for gastrojejunostomy tube.
- Peelaway sheath may be inserted.
- Tube inserted into proximal jejunum and held in place with either intragastric balloon or intragastric locking loop.
- Some tubes are best placed over a stiff hydrophilic wire.

Follow-Up

Patients should ideally be seen regularly in a dedicated gastrostomy clinic where the following can be assessed:
- Stoma and tube condition
- Nutritional state and feeding regime
- Weight

Alternative Therapies

Endoscopic Gastrostomy

- This requires more sedation.
- Has a higher complication rate.
- Should not be performed in patients with oropharyngeal cancer due to risk of tumor seeding to gastrostomy site and also for obvious mechanical reasons.

Complications

Tube misplacement (within tract or peritoneum):

- Measure tract correctly
- Maintain forward pressure while inflating balloon

Colon perforation:

- Should never occur with radiological gastrostomy
- Ensure colon is visible, if collapsed use ultrasound to check

Liver perforation:

- Always palpate liver edge or use ultrasound to check

T fastener placement in posterior stomach wall:

- Can occur if stomach not well inflated particularly with antral punctures
- Check anterior wall and not posterior wall is pulled when you tug on the T fastener
- Cut T fastener at skin and place another one if this occurs

Tube falling out:

- Do not remove T fasteners if this occurs while they are in situ.
- If within first few days replace tube under screening control.
- Long-standing stomas should have a new tube placed immediately even if just a Foley catheter as tract will rapidly close up.

Key Points

> Choose correct type of tube
> Percutaneous (not per oral) in oropharyngeal cancer patients
> Ensure adequate gastric distension
> Use gastropexy
> Measure tract length correctly
> Maintain forward pressure during balloon inflation
> Check tube positioned correctly

Suggested Reading

A video of this procedure may be seen online in the video section of Which medical Device.com
http://www.whichmedicaldevice.com

1. Wollman B, D'Agostino HB, Walus-Wigle JR, Easter DW, Beale A. Radiologic, endoscopic, and surgical gastrostomy: an institutional evaluation and meta-analysis of the literature. *Radiology*. 1995;197(3):699-704.
2. Thornton FJ, Varghese JC, Haslam PJ, Mc Grath FP, Keeling F, Lee MJ. Percutaneous gastrostomy in patients who fail or are unsuitable for endoscopic gastrostomy. *CVIR*. 2000;23(4): 279-284.
3. Thornton FJ, Fotheringham T, Haslam PJ, Mc Grath FP, Keeling F, Lee MJ. Percutaneous radiologic gastrostomy with and without T-fastener gastropexy: A Randomised Comparison Study. *Cardovascul Intervent Radiol*. 2002;25:467-471.
4. Lyon SM, Haslam PJ, Duke DM, McGrath FP, Lee MJ. De novo placement of button gastrostomy catheters in an adult population: experience in 53 patients. *J Vasc Interv Radiol*. 2003;14(10):1283-1289.

Index